Current Management of Foot and Ankle Trauma

Guest Editor

MICHAEL P. CLARE, MD

FOOT AND ANKLE CLINICS

www.foot.theclinics.com

Consulting Editor
MARK S. MYERSON, MD

December 2008 • Volume 13 • Number 4

SAUNDERS an imprint of ELSEVIER, Inc.

W.B. SAUNDERS COMPANY
A Division of Elsevier Inc.

1600 John F. Kennedy Blvd. • Suite 1800 • Philadelphia, PA 19103-2899

http://www.theclinics.com

FOOT AND ANKLE CLINICS Volume 13, Number 4
December 2008 ISSN 1083-7515, ISBN-10: 1-4160-6296-3, ISBN-13: 978-1-4160-6296-7

Editor: Debora Dellapena

Photocopying
Single photocopies of single articles may be made for personal use as allowed by national copyright laws. Permission of the Publisher and payment of a fee is required for all other photocopying, including multiple or systematic copying, copying for advertising or promotional purposes, resale, and all forms of document delivery. Special rates are available for educational institutions that wish to make photocopies for non-profit educational classroom use. For information on how to seek permission visit www.elsevier.com/permissions or call: (+44) 1865 843830 (UK)/(+1) 215 239 3804 (USA).

Derivative Works
Subscribers may reproduce tables of contents or prepare lists of articles including abstracts for internal circulation within their institutions. Permission of the Publisher is required for resale or distribution outside the institution. Permission of the Publisher is required for all other derivative works, including compilations and translations (please consult www.elsevier.com/permissions).

Electronic Storage or Usage
Permission of the Publisher is required to store or use electronically any material contained in this journal, including any article or part of an article (please consult www.elsevier.com/permissions). Except as outlined above, no part of this publication may be reproduced, stored in a retrieval system or transmitted in any form or by any means, electronic, mechanical, photocopying, recording or otherwise, without prior written permission of the Publisher.

Notice
No responsibility is assumed by the Publisher for any injury and/or damage to persons or property as a matter of products liability, negligence or otherwise, or from any use or operation of any methods, products, instructions or ideas contained in the material herein. Because of rapid advances in the medical sciences, in particular, independent verification of diagnoses and drug dosages should be made.

Although all advertising material is expected to conform to ethical (medical) standards, inclusion in this publication does not constitute a guarantee or endorsement of the quality or value of such product or of the claims made by its manufacturer.

Foot and Ankle Clinics (ISSN 1083-7515) is published quarterly by Elsevier, Inc., 360 Park Avenue South, New York, NY 10010-1710. Months of issue are March, June, September, and December. Business and Editorial Offices: 1600 John F. Kennedy Blvd., Suite 1800, Philadelphia, PA 19103-2899. Customer Service Office: 11830 Westline Industrial Drive, St. Louis, MO 63146. Periodicals postage paid at New York, NY, and additional mailing offices. Subscription price per year is $230.00 (US individuals), $333.00 (US institutions), $116.00 (US students), $257.00 (Canadian individuals), $394.00 (Canadian institutions), $159.00 (Canadian students), $331.00 (foreign individuals), $394.00 (foreign institutions), and $159.00 (foreign students). To receive student/resident rate, orders must be accompanied by name of affiliated institution, date of term, and the *signature* of program/residency coordinator on institution letterhead. Orders will be billed at individual rate until proof of status is received. Foreign air speed delivery is included in all *Clinics* subscription prices. All prices are subject to change without notice. **POSTMASTER:** Send address changes to *Foot and Ankle Clinics*, Elsevier Periodicals Customer Service, 11830 Westline Industrial Drive, St. Louis, MO 63146. **Customer Service: 1-800-654-2452 (US). From outside of the United States, call 314-453-7041. Fax: 314-453-5170. E-mail: JournalsCustomerService-usa@elsevier.com (for print support); JournalsOnlineSupport-usa@elsevier. com (for online support).**

Reprints. For copies of 100 or more, of articles in this publication, please contact the Commercial Reprints Department, Elsevier Inc., 360 Park Avenue South, New York, NY 10010-1710. Tel.: 212-633-3812; Fax: 212-462-1935; E-mail: reprints@elsevier.com.

Printed in the United States of America.

Contributors

CONSULTING EDITOR

MARK S. MYERSON, MD
Director, Institute for Foot and Ankle Reconstruction at Mercy, Mercy Medical Center, Baltimore, Maryland

GUEST EDITOR

MICHAEL P. CLARE, MD
Director of Fellowship Education, Foot and Ankle Fellowship, Florida Orthopaedic Institute, Tampa, Florida

AUTHORS

DAVID P. BAREI, MD, FRCS(C)
Associate Professor, Department of Orthopaedics and Sports Medicine, Harborview Medical Center, University of Washington, Seattle, Washington

JENNIFER M.B. BREY, MD
Department of Orthopaedic Surgery, Drexel College of Medicine, Philadelphia, Pennsylvania

MICHAEL D. CASTRO, DO
The Center for Orthopaedic Research and Education, Phoenix, Arizona

MICHAEL P. CLARE, MD
Director of Fellowship Education, Foot and Ankle Fellowship, Florida Orthopaedic Institute, Tampa, Florida

J. CHRIS COETZEE, MD
Minnesota Sports Medicine and Twin Cities Orthopedics; and Adjunct Associate Professor, Department of Orthopedics, University of Minnesota, Eden Prairie, Minnesota

JOHN S. EARLY, MD
Clinical Professor of Orthopaedic Surgery, University of Texas Southwestern Medical Center; Texas Orthopaedic Associates LLP, Dallas, Texas

RENÉ GRASS, MD, PhD
Professor of Trauma Surgery; Attending Trauma Surgeon, Klinik und Poliklinik für Unfall, Wiederherstellungschirurgie Universitätsklinikum, "Carl Gustav Carus" der TU Dresden, Dresden, Germany

G. YVES LAFLAMME, MD
Assistant Professor, Department of Orthopaedic Surgery, Université de Montréal, Hôspital Sacré-Coeur de Montréal, Quebec, Canada

STEPHANE LÉDUC, MD
Assistant Professor, Department of Orthopaedic Surgery, Université de Montréal, Hôspital Sacré-Coeur de Montréal, Quebec, Canada

MATTHEW A. MORMINO, MD
Associate Professor, Department of Orthopaedic Surgery and Rehabilitation, University of Nebraska Medical Center, Omaha, Nebraska

MARK S. MYERSON, MD
Director, Institute for Foot and Ankle Reconstruction at Mercy, Mercy Medical Center, Baltimore, Maryland

SCOTT NEMEC, DO
Orthopedic Resident, Department of Medical Education, Ingham Regional Medical Center, Michigan State University College of Osteopathic Medicine, Lansing Michigan

SEAN E. NORK, MD
Associate Professor, Department of Orthopaedics and Sports Medicine, Harborview Medical Center, University of Washington, Seattle, Washington

HANS-CHRISTOPH PAPE, MD
Division Chief, Orthopedic Trauma, University of Pittsburgh Medical Center, Division of Orthopedic Trauma, Pittsburgh, Pennsylvania

ANTHONY PERERA, MBChB FRCS(Orth)
Foot and Ankle Fellow, Institute for Foot and Ankle Reconstruction at Mercy, Mercy Medical Center, Baltimore, Maryland

STEFAN RAMMELT, MD, PhD
Lecturer in Trauma Surgery; Attending Trauma Surgeon, Klinik und Poliklinik für Unfall, Wiederherstellungschirurgie Universitätsklinikum, "Carl Gustav Carus" der TU Dresden, Dresden, Germany

LORI K. REED, MD
Assistant Professor of Orthopaedic Surgery, Department of Orthopaedic Surgery and Rehabilitation, University of Nebraska Medical Center, Omaha, Nebraska

ROY W. SANDERS, MD
Director, Orthopaedic Trauma Service, Tampa General Hospital, The Florida Orthopaedic Institute, Tampa, Florida

MATTHEW SCHRAMSKI, DO
Orthopedic Resident, Department of Medical Education, Ingham Regional Medical Center, Michigan State University College of Osteopathic Medicine, Lansing, Michigan

AARON SOP, DO
Orthopedic Trauma Fellow, University of Pittsburgh Medical Center, Division of Orthopedic Trauma, Pittsburgh, Pennsylvania

SCOTT A. SWANSON, MD
Nebraska Orthopaedics and Sports Medicine, St. Elizabeth Medical Plaza, Lincoln, Nebraska

KYLE SWITZER, DO
Orthopedic Resident, Department of Medical Education, Ingham Regional Medical Center, Michigan State University College of Osteopathic Medicine, Lansing Michigan

MICHAEL P. SWORDS, DO
Assistant Clinical Professor, Michigan State University College of Osteopathic Medicine, Section of Orthopedics, Sparrow Health System, Mid Michigan Orthopaedic Institute, East Lansing, Michigan

IVAN S. TARKIN, MD
Assistant Professor, Department of Orthopaedic Surgery, University of Pittsburgh Medical Center, Pittsburgh, Pennsylvania

ARTHUR K. WALLING, MD
Florida Orthopaedic Institute, Tampa, Florida

HANS ZWIPP, MD, PhD
Professor of Trauma Surgery; Chief of the Department of Trauma and Reconstructive Surgery, Klinik und Poliklinik für Unfall, Wiederherstellungschirurgie Universitätsklinikum, "Carl Gustav Carus" der TU Dresden, Dresden, Germany

Contents

Preface xiii

Michael P. Clare

Fractures of the Tibial Plafond 571

David P. Barei and Sean E. Nork

> High-energy fractures of the tibial plafond are a lifechanging event for the patient. Currently, open reduction and internal fixation (ORIF) appears to offer the best chance for obtaining and maintaining anatomic articular reduction and axial alignment to union. Definitive ORIF should be performed in a staged fashion to allow adequate resolution of the associated soft tissue injury. A preoperative plan is essential to a successful outcome and it must include a strategy to access and stabilize the articular and nonarticular components of the injury.

A Rational Approach to Ankle Fractures 593

Michael P. Clare

> Ankle fractures involve a spectrum of injury patterns from simple to complex, such that these injuries are not always "just an ankle fracture." By combining the injury mechanism and the radiographic findings, the surgeon can apply the Lauge-Hansen classification in taking a rational approach to the management of these fractures.

Injuries to the Distal Tibiofibular Syndesmosis: An Evidence-Based Approach to Acute and Chronic Lesions 611

Stefan Rammelt, Hans Zwipp, and René Grass

> Injuries to the distal tibiofibular syndesmosis are frequent in collision sports. Most of these injuries are not associated with latent or frank diastasis between the distal tibia and fibula and are treated as high ankle sprains, with an extended protocol of physical therapy. Relevant instability of the syndesmosis results from rupture of two or more ligaments leading to a diastasis of more than 2 mm and requiring surgical fixation. Most of these syndesmosis ruptures are associated with bony avulsions or malleolar fractures. Treatment consists of anatomic reduction of the fibula and fixation with one or two tibiofibular syndesmosis screws. Proper reduction and positioning of the screws are more predictive of a good clinical result than the material, size, and number of cortices purchased. Chronic injuries without instability are treated by arthroscopic or open debridement and arthrolysis. Chronic syndesmotic instability can be treated with

a three-strand peroneus longus ligamentoplasty in the absence of symptomatic arthritis or bony defects.

Talus Fracture Management   635

John S. Early

Talar head and fracture injuries are not easily recognized and can create significant long-term disability when missed. Careful investigation of any injury about the ankle requires both clinical and radiographic examination. A computed tomography scan is extremely helpful in diagnosing and treating talus fractures. Displaced fractures require open reduction of the major joint surfaces and internal fixation. Prolonged non–weight bearing and immobilization is the norm. Despite aggressive management, complications involving avascular necrosis and posttraumatic arthritis to both the subtalar and tibiotalar joints occurs frequently.

Management of Intra-Articular Fractures of the Calcaneus   659

Scott A. Swanson, Michael P. Clare, and Roy W. Sanders

The majority of calcaneal fractures are intra-articular fractures resulting from high-energy trauma. Many of these occur in young men in their prime working years and result in significant loss of economic productivity. Surgical treatment generally is indicated for displaced, intra-articular fractures. Open reduction and internal fixation through an extensile lateral incision is the mainstay of surgical approaches and has provided consistent results. Minimally invasive techniques are now emerging and new technology, such as locking plates and intraoperative 3-D fluoroscopy, may aid orthopedic surgeons who treat these difficult fractures.

Chopart Fractures and Dislocations   679

Michael P. Swords, Matthew Schramski, Kyle Switzer, and Scott Nemec

Fractures and dislocations of the midfoot and Chopart complex are among the most difficult foot injuries to manage. The treating surgeon is faced with a wide array of treatment challenges. Plain radiographs often grossly underestimate the extent of injury. The anatomy in this region of the foot is quite intricate with numerous articulations. Fractures can occur in isolation or as part of a more complex injury pattern. Misdiagnosis and under treatment can lead to severe alterations of both normal anatomy and function. This article discusses the rationales and techniques for treating these difficult injuries.

Making Sense of Lisfranc Injuries 695

J. Chris Coetzee

Management of Lisfranc injuries has evoked significant debate and controversy over the years, and there is no indication that the controversy is nearing an end. Probably the main reason for the controversy is because a "Lisfranc injury" is part of a very wide and poorly defined spectrum of injuries. Not all Lisfranc injuries are created equal, and there will never be a single treatment option for all these injuries. Lisfranc injuries are relatively uncommon, but if undetected, untreated or under-treated can cause morbidity and disability. The objective of this article is to provide guidelines for treatment of the spectrum of Lisfranc injuries.

High-Energy Foot and Ankle Trauma: Principles for Formulating an Individualized Care Plan 705

Ivan S. Tarkin, Aaron Sop, and Hans-Christoph Pape

Care of the patient with high-energy foot and ankle trauma requires an individualized care plan. Staged treatment respecting the traumatized soft tissue envelope is often advisable. Wound care is a priority, and the vacuum-assisted closure dressing serves an integral role. Before definitive reconstruction, the surgeon needs to develop a treatment plan designed to match the unique personality of the patient and injury. Amputation is considered a rational treatment option for the patient with severe injury and poor host biology. Despite the most appropriate management, many severe foot and ankle injuries have a guarded prognosis.

Distal Tibia Nonunions 725

Lori K. Reed and Matthew A. Mormino

Although tibia metaphyseal nonunion is rare, its treatment is often complex. The merits of related management techniques are discussed. These techniques include: intramedullary nailing, fine wire fixation, and blade plate reconstruction, which is the method preferred by the authors.

Surgical Techniques for the Reconstruction of Malunited Ankle Fractures 737

Anthony Perera and Mark Myerson

Ankle fractures are so common and most heal well so there is a certain lack of attention for the potential for adverse consequences and the potential to salvage these complications. There is a clear association between ankle fracture malunion and a poor outcome, whilst reconstruction can often be accomplished it can be very difficult. The key lies in accurate assessment, careful preoperative planning and proficiency in specialised reconstructive techniques. In this article, we describe this process using clinical cases to illustrate the management of malunion.

Posttraumatic Avascular Necrosis of theTalus   753

Stephane Léduc, Michael P. Clare, G. Yves Laflamme, and Arthur K. Walling

> Avascular necrosis of the talus is one the most challenging problems encountered in posttraumatic reconstruction of the hindfoot. Since the first description of the talus injury in 1608 by Fabricius of Hilden, our knowledge of the talar anatomy, injuries, sequelae, and management has increased significantly. Adequate knowledge of the etiology, the extent of the disease, and the degree of patient symptoms are required to determine optimal treatment.

Salvage of Compartment Syndrome of the Leg and Foot   767

Jennifer M.B. Brey and Michael D. Castro

> Early diagnosis and treatment of compartment syndrome of the leg or foot is invaluable in avoiding a chronic and often debilitating course. In cases where an ischemic contracture results in pain, disability or soft tissue compromise, surgical intervention is indicated. Thorough physical examination of patients and a thorough understanding of pathomechanics of the foot and ankle are paramount. These combined with a comprehensive preoperative plan and meticulous execution can often provide improved function and decrease pain in patients affected by this debilitating problem.

Index   773

FORTHCOMING ISSUES

March 2009
The Hallux
John Campbell, MD, *Guest Editor*

June 2009
Complex Injuries of the Foot and Ankle
in Sport
David Porter, MD, PhD, *Guest Editor*

September 2009
Correction of Multiplanar Deformity of the
Foot and Ankle
Anish R. Kadakia, MD, *Guest Editor*

December 2009
Achilles Tendon
Drew Murphy, MD, *Guest Editor*

RECENT ISSUES

September 2008
Ankle Arthritis
Steven M. Raikin, MD, *Guest Editor*

June 2008
Cavovarus Foot
John S. Early, MD, *Guest Editor*

March 2008
External Fixation for Lower Limb Salvage
Paul Cooper, MD, *Guest Editor*

THE CLINICS ARE NOW AVAILABLE ONLINE!

Access your subscription at:
www.theclinics.com

Preface

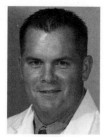

Michael P. Clare, MD
Guest Editor

Foot and ankle trauma remains an area of considerable challenge to both the ortho-paedic trauma surgeon and the orthopaedic foot and ankle surgeon. The limited soft tissue envelope coupled with a high concentration of force across relatively small joints produces injuries associated with substantial long-term morbidity. Continued develop-ments in surgical techniques and specific, anatomically contoured implants have led to improved treatment outcomes and functional results. This issue of *Foot and Ankle Clinics* includes contributions from several well-respected foot and ankle trauma surgeons, and focuses on current strategies in the management of foot and ankle trauma and post-trauma reconstruction.

Michael P. Clare, MD
Director of Fellowship Education
Foot and Ankle Fellowship
Florida Orthopaedic Institute
13020 Telecom Parkway North
Tampa, FL 33637, USA

E-mail address:
mpclare@verizon.net (M.P. Clare)

Foot Ankle Clin N Am 13 (2008) xiii
doi:10.1016/j.fcl.2008.09.007
1083-7515/08/$ – see front matter © 2008 Elsevier Inc. All rights reserved.

foot.theclinics.com

Fractures of the Tibial Plafond

David P. Barei, MD, FRCS(C)*, Sean E. Nork, MD

KEYWORDS

• Pilon • Plafond • Fracture • Distal tibia • Staged treatment

Fractures involving the distal tibia remain one of the most considerable therapeutic challenges that confront the orthopaedic traumatologist. Numerous features of these injuries are responsible for this, but none are as troublesome as the associated soft tissue injury that is frequently present. The evolution of the surgical management of distal tibia fractures has progressed over the past thirty years in large part due to an improved understanding of the importance of the soft tissue envelope. Specifically, the orthopaedic community has discovered that re-establishing the osseous anatomy while ignoring the soft tissue envelope frequently leads to suboptimal postoperative results and high complication rates. Although multiple treatment approaches have been described, there is no consensus regarding the optimal treatment of these injuries, and long-term outcome data from randomized comparative treatment methods remains lacking.

Intra-articular fractures of the distal tibial weight-bearing surface are usually the result of rotational or axial loading forces. These two main mechanisms of injury result in significantly different fracture patterns, soft tissue damage, associated injuries, and prognosis. Associated fibular fractures are common to both injury mechanisms.

Intra-articular distal tibia fractures resulting from rotational forces have a spiral orientation, frequently without significant fracture comminution. The articular injury is composed of mildly or moderately displaced large articular fragments with minimal chondral impaction or disruption. The soft tissue envelope is injured to a lesser degree, although significant swelling may still be a component. Open wounds with significant devitalization are not common. The prognosis is more favorable than with axial-loading injuries.[1]

Axial-loading injuries to the tibial plafond frequently result from motor vehicle collisions or falls from significant heights. From the French language, the term "pilon" was introduced by Destot in 1911; it refers to a pestle, which is a club-shaped tool for mashing, or grinding substances in a mortar or a large bar moved vertically to stamp or pound. Though commonly used interchangeably with the term "plafond," a pilon fracture is a descriptive term suggesting that the talus acts as a hammer, or pestle,

Department of Orthopaedics and Sports Medicine, Harborview Medical Center, University of Washington, 325 Ninth Avenue, Box 359798 -Rm 6EC21, Seattle, WA 98104, USA
* Corresponding author.
E-mail address: jbould@u.washington.edu (D.P. Barei).

Foot Ankle Clin N Am 13 (2008) 571–591
doi:10.1016/j.fcl.2008.09.002

foot.theclinics.com

that impacts and injures the tibial plafond. The advent of high-speed motor vehicle travel, improved automotive restraint systems, and improved life-saving trauma care systems have resulted in the increased incidence of axial load-type intra-articular distal tibia fractures that confront the orthopaedist. These injuries may present in isolation but are more frequently seen in the polytraumatized patient. Marked articular and metaphyseal comminution, wide displacement, chondral impaction, and articular debris are commonly seen. Open wounds, deep abrasions, fracture blisters, compartmental syndromes, and accompanying osseous and soft tissue devitalization are common and corroborate the high-energy mechanism. The ultimate fracture pattern depends on the direction and rate of application of the injuries force, and on the position of the foot at the time of loading. High-energy axial loading injuries have a worse prognosis.[2–4]

ASSESSMENT
Physical Examination

Examination of the soft tissue envelope is of critical importance in the complete assessment of fractures of the tibial plafond and should be performed in a logical, consistent, and circumferential manner. The degree of swelling, the severity of contusions, and the presence of abrasions, blisters, open wounds, and compartmental syndrome are evaluated and noted. Not infrequently, widely displaced fracture fragments may create excessive skin tension and jeopardize local skin circulation. In these situations, manual correction of these gross deformities must be performed expeditiously, before radiographic examination, to minimize further vascular compromise to the local skin and soft tissues. The circulatory status is evaluated by palpation and/or Doppler ultrasound examination of the pedal pulses, and by noting the color and temperature of the foot. The dorsal and plantar aspects of the foot are examined for alterations in sensation. Open wounds are treated with initiation of intravenous antibiotics, removal of obvious foreign material and debris, sterile saline irrigation, and coverage with a sterile bandage. Occasionally, a fragment of bone remains extruded through the skin, resulting in crushing of the underlying skin and soft tissue envelope. Frequently, this scenario occurs when the distal portion of the tibial shaft is extruded through the anteromedial skin of the distal tibia, putting the skin at the distal portion of the wound in jeopardy. In this situation, reduction of the extruded fragment should be attempted with the goal being to relieve further injury to the anteromedial soft tissues. After the limb has been evaluated, it is re-aligned and placed it into a provisional splint that does not obscure radiographic detail.

Radiographic Examination

Initial anteroposterior (AP), mortise, and lateral radiographs are obtained. Full-length images of the tibia and fibula complete the radiological examination of the injured leg. The diagnosis of a displaced fracture of the tibial plafond is made on these radiographs. The presence and location of an associated fibular fracture, the degree of articular disruption, and the direction of displacement of the talus and associated fracture fragments are important fracture characteristics to note.

Computerized tomography (CT) improves the ability to assess the injury and to formulate a preoperative plan before definitive fixation.[5] Thin cut axial images combined with coronal and sagittal reformatting allow evaluation of major fracture planes, articular impaction, and the degree of comminution. To optimize comprehension of fracture relationships, however, CT scanning should be performed after a provisional reduction is obtained. CT scans obtained with substantial shortening, angulation, and displacements of the limb and fracture fragments make the identification of fracture details more difficult and render formulation of a preoperative surgical plan suboptimal.

There are occasions, however, when acute CT scanning of the distal tibia is appropriate. Invariably, this situation occurs when the plain radiographs demonstrate a "simple" and modestly displaced articular injury with a soft tissue envelope that does not preclude early open reduction and internal fixation (ORIF), or as part of a seemingly extra-articular distal tibia fracture with plain radiographic clues that suggest an intra-articular extension. In this latter situation, the CT scan is used as a diagnostic tool. The distinguishing features of these two scenarios are: first, that the interpretation of the CT scan is comprehensible; and second, in the setting of a satisfactory soft tissue envelope, the operative strategy may consist of a single stage surgical procedure.

TREATMENT
Nonoperative Treatment

Nonoperative management should be reserved for those fractures that are truly non-displaced or for those patients that have a significant or absolute contraindication to surgical management. Patients treated using nonoperative methods can be effectively managed with closed manipulative reduction and cast immobilization. Progressive weight-bearing with ankle and subtalar range of motion is initiated based on radiographic healing. Indications for nonoperative management of displaced intra-articular fractures of the tibial plafond are extremely limited.

Casting is ineffective in maintaining limb length and in reducing impacted articular segments. In those intra-articular distal tibia fractures with an intact fibula, the persistent varus tendency makes maintenance of limb alignment with nonoperative techniques difficult. Similarly, displaced partial articular injuries frequently demonstrate talar subluxation within the mortise that cannot be effectively managed with closed techniques. Despite the shortcomings of closed treatment, this management method is preferred in a number of patients, including those that are bedridden or that have minimal ambulatory capacity or functional demands. Additionally, patients with significant associated medical comorbidities, particularly those that substantially affect bone and soft tissue healing may be candidates for closed treatment.

Operative Treatment

The majority of displaced distal tibial fractures are managed operatively, particularly those injuries with displaced intra-articular fracture fragments. Unstable, displaced, extra-articular distal tibial fractures can be treated with numerous techniques including: external fixation, open reduction and plate fixation, percutaneous or indirect reduction with minimally invasive plate fixation, medullary nailing, and combinations thereof. The fracture pattern and conditions of the local soft tissue envelope are the major determinants for choosing the surgical technique.

The tibiotalar joint poorly tolerates articular incongruity and talar subluxation. The degree to which residual articular incongruity affects long-term functional outcomes, post-traumatic arthrosis, and the need for further surgical intervention, however, remains controversial. Although there are no strict guidelines for determining how much articular step-off or gap can be tolerated, a visible incongruity at the tibial plafond that is demonstrated on plain radiographs should be considered an indication for operative reduction and fixation in properly selected patients. Associated angular malalignment and/or talar subluxation further jeopardize tibiotalar joint function, especially with associated articular incongruity, and they are strong indications for operative management.

General Approach to Open Reduction and Internal Fixation

After a thorough evaluation of patient, soft tissue, and fracture characteristics, a formal surgical tactic can begin to be formulated. The principles described by Ruedi and Allogower[6,7] over 20 years ago remain a solid foundation and continue to guide many current treatment decisions. The original description of these four principles consisted of: restoration of anatomic fibular length, anatomic restoration of the distal tibial articular surface, bone grafting of metaphyseal defects, and stable fixation of the fracture with medial buttress plating. Although some flexibility is required when managing these challenging injuries, these basic principles remain the foundation for formulating a surgical tactic.

Over the last two decades, however, the orthopaedic community has learned that the application of these principles in the absence of an understanding of the associated soft tissue injury and/or in the absence of meticulous soft tissue handling resulted in disastrous complications.[8,9] Improvements in soft tissue handling, the use of lower profile implants, and the use of percutaneous and limited incision exposures have all contributed to decreasing significant wound complication rates. Perhaps the most significant factors that have resulted in decreasing wound complications are the recognition of the soft tissue injury and the development of a surgical tactic that considers timing and soft tissue recovery. Most surgeons currently favor a two-stage protocol designed to promote recovery of the traumatized soft tissue envelope before definitive fixation.[10,11] Currently, the initial or first stage of displaced tibial pilon fracture management focuses on stabilization of the soft tissue envelope. The subsequent or second stage of management is devoted to the definitive reduction and stabilization of the articular surface and axial alignment.

Stage 1: Urgent Surgical Management

The components of the first stage are focused primarily on stabilization of the soft tissue envelope. This is performed as an urgent surgical procedure as soon as the patient's general condition permits. The key components of this stage include: the anticipation of all skin incisions; debridement of any open wounds; a four-compartment fasciotomy if required; ORIF of the fibular fracture if present; and reduction and temporary spanning external fixation of the tibial plafond fracture. In a small subset of tibial pilon fracture patterns, extension of the fracture may propagate into the diaphysis. Occasionally, acute reduction and stabilization of this fracture component may facilitate the subsequent stage of definitive articular and axial reductions and fixations.[12]

Fibular ORIF and tibial external fixation

If fractured, fibular reduction and stabilization is an integral part of the initial management of these injuries for several reasons. First, restoration of accurate fibular length, alignment and rotation indirectly reduces the majority of tibial deformity secondary to the ligamentous and other soft tissue attachments between the two bones. Second, the remainder of residual tibial displacement can be managed with a medially based ankle joint spanning external fixator using the reduced and stabilized fibula as a fulcrum for the external fixator. Third, anatomic reduction of the fibula facilitates indirect reduction of the associated anterior (Chaput) and posterior (Volkmann) tibial articular fragments via the anterior and posterior distal tibiofibular syndesmotic ligaments, respectively.[13] Fibular reduction usually neutralizes the tendency for valgus angulation and/or lateral translation of the talus and associated tibial pilon fracture fragments.

Unlike the relatively simple fibular fractures seen in rotational ankle fractures involving the malleoli, the fibular fractures seen with tibial pilon fractures are frequently comminuted with transverse and oblique fracture plane orientations. Because of this, the surgeon should choose fibular implants based upon the degree of comminution and the degree to which they will provide fracture stability. One-third tubular plates are a common choice, but stiffer constructs, such as stacked one-third tubular plates, pre-contoured distal fibular peri-articular plates and 2.7 mm or 3.5 mm dynamic compression plates, may be required.

Invariably, the optimal incision for reduction and fixation of the fibula is posterior to the palpable posterolateral border of the fibula. The fascia overlying the peroneal musculature (lateral compartment) is incised and the peroneus longus and brevis muscles are retracted posteriorly. The fibula is reduced using direct or indirect techniques, or a combination thereof, and stabilizing implants are typically applied to the posterolateral aspect of the fibula.[14,15] The benefits of the posterolateral incision for fixation of the fibula include: preservation of an adequate skin bridge for subsequent anterior or anterolateral surgical approaches to the distal tibia;[16] minimization of fibular soft tissue complications because the incision is not directly over the subcutaneous portion of the fibula; and facilitation of access to the posterolateral aspect of the tibial plafond with elevation of the peronei anteriorly and elevation of the flexor hallucis longus musculature from the posterior aspect of the tibia.[17,18]

The application of temporary spanning external fixation of the tibial plafond is usually performed after fibular stabilization. External fixation effectively stabilizes the tibial component of the injury, maintains neutral talar tilt, and resists the tendency of the talus to displace anteriorly out of the tibial plafond. Closed manipulation and spanning external fixation achieves these goals indirectly using ligamentotaxis, and allows soft tissue recovery by stabilizing the underlying skeleton. In the setting of an intact fibula or a surgically stabilized fibula, a medially-based frame is typically employed. A uniplanar 5.0-mm Schanz pin is placed from anteromedial to posterolateral through the tibial diaphysis followed by a second 5.0-mm pin from medial to lateral into the calcaneal tuberosity. Placement of the calcaneal Schanz pin is in the posterior aspect of the calcaneal tuberosity and should avoid the numerous calcaneal sensory branches from the tibial nerve.[19] A 4.0-mm Schanz pin is placed from medial to lateral across the three cuneiforms of the ipsilateral midfoot. To minimize the risk of septic complications after definitive surgery, these pins are inserted well out of the anticipated location of plates, screws, and incisions. Manipulating the calcaneal Shanz pin typically performs the vast majority of the reduction. The usual reduction maneuvers applied to the hindfoot are traction (restoring tibial length), varus or valgus correction (to achieve a horizontal talar dome), and posterior translation (correcting the commonly seen anterior displacement). After tibial length, alignment, and rotation are restored, a radiolucent bar connecting the tibial pin to the calcaneal pin is applied. Placing this initial bar stabilizes the vast majority of the reduction. At this point, the talus should be centered beneath the tibia on both the AP and lateral fluoroscopic images, and the articular surface of the talus should be perpendicular to the longitudinal axis of the tibial shaft. Accurate return of length is estimated by re-establishing the normal relationship of the lateral process of the talus with the distal tip of the fibula.[20] Because the bar is located posterior to the mechanical axis of the tibia, the talus is maintained posteriorly beneath the tibial plafond and out of the typical anterior displacement. Subsequently, a tibial to cuneiform bar is placed to maintain neutral dorsi- and plantar-flexion of the tibiotalar joint. A third bar is used to connect the calcaneal pin to the cuneiform pin thereby neutralizing forefoot adduction and to increase the rigidity of the external fixation construct. A second 5.0-mm anteromedial to posterolateral Schanz pin is placed into the tibial diaphysis and connected to both of the vertically-oriented bars, finalizing the construct (**Fig. 1**).

In situations where the fibula is not amenable to acute ORIF, such as secondary to poor local soft tissue conditions, fracture complexity, or other patient factors, a biplanar external fixator is employed. The essential features distinguishing this frame from the medially-based frame described above are the use of a trans-calcaneal Schanz pin and the placement of the tibial diaphyseal pins in a more anterior to posterior direction rather than anteromedial to posterolateral. The calcaneal Schanz pin is manipulated using both the lateral and medial pin extensions from the calcaneus. Because the fibula is unstable, manipulation of the calcaneus from both the medial and lateral aspects substantially improves the ability to control the coronal alignment of the distal tibia. Two bars are used to secure the tibial pin(s) to the calcaneal pin: one medially and one laterally. The remainder of the construct is similar to that described for the medially based frame. In addition to the unstabilized fibula, the authors' main indications for the use of a transcalcaneal Schanz pin external fixation construct are: (1) tibial pilon fractures with a delayed presentation (greater than one week post-injury); or (2) tibial pilon fractures that demonstrate substantial valgus angulation despite an intact or operatively reduced and stabilized fibula (**Fig. 2** A–D). The fibular incision is closed using a modified Allgower-Donati suture[21] with the knots tied posteriorly, and the limb is placed into a well-padded splint. A CT scan of the tibial plafond is then obtained to aid in planning definitive fixation. Definitive reduction and fixation is typically performed 7–21 days later and only after soft tissue recovery has occurred.[10,11]

Stage 2: Definitive Surgical Management

Definitive management of the high-energy tibial pilon fracture is challenging, and the optimal method of reduction and fixation remains controversial.[22–24] The historically high incidence of serious wound complications associated with traditional open methods has popularized minimally invasive reduction and stabilization techniques.[25–29] Limited arthrotomy with percutaneous management of the articular injury, combined with the use of fine wire or hybrid external fixation to neutralize meta-diaphyseal comminution may reduce the incidence of deep wound sepsis by minimizing soft tissue disruption. Nevertheless, obtaining and maintaining a satisfactory articular reduction with these techniques is difficult. Restoration of the articular surface along with stable fixation allows early motion and has been felt to be the most important predictor of satisfactory outcome,[2–4,7,30] although this is controversial.[31] Open management, however, must be performed with meticulous attention to preoperative planning, soft tissue handling, and the appropriate timing of intervention. If soft tissue complications can be avoided, anatomic articular reduction with stable fixation maximizes the chance of obtaining a satisfactory outcome.[9]

Fracture anatomy

An understanding the tibial plafond fracture anatomy is useful in allowing the surgeon to develop a surgical tactic for definitive surgical management. Despite the numerous possibilities, certain reproducible elements can be identified. Partial articular injuries (Orthopaedic Trauma Association [OTA] B-Type) commonly involve disruption of either the medial malleolus or the anterior plafond. Despite being seemingly less severe than their OTA C-Type counterparts (**Figs. 3** and **4**), these B-type injuries will frequently display articular crushing and impaction of the osteochondral surface immediately adjacent to the leading edge of the intact segment.

Because the ligamentous structures of the ankle remain largely intact after a tibial pilon fracture, OTA C-Type injury patterns commonly demonstrate three main fracture segments: the anterolateral (Chaput) fragment; the posterior (Volkmann) fragment; and the medial malleolar fragment (See **Fig. 2** E). Each of these fragments, in turn, remains attached to the anterior tibiofibular ligament, the posterior tibiofibular ligament, and the deltoid ligament, respectively. Topliss and colleagues have noted that the major fracture patterns can be categorized in two discrete groups based on the primary fracture plane orientations: the sagittal plane or the coronal plane.[32] The sagittal plane fractures tended to present in varus, had more proximal metadiaphyseal disruption, and followed a higher energy injury in younger adults. The coronal fracture patterns tended to present in valgus, had a more distal dissociation, and followed lower energy trauma in older patients.

Comminution is frequently identified along the fracture lines separating the major articular components. The preoperative plan includes an assessment of the major fracture components and how their manipulation will allow access to the areas of comminution, while respecting their soft tissue and ligamentous attachments. A rational choice for stabilizing implants will allow the reduced articular fragments to be secured and neutralize the major displacing forces that occur in the metadiaphyseal region.

Surgical exposures

Modified anteromedial approach The anteromedial approach is an extensile exposure that allows wide visualization of the anterior and medial aspects of the tibial plafond. The traditional anteromedial approach described by the AO Group[33] uses the classic anteromedial incision, which parallels the course of the tibialis anterior tendon but generally does not allow for complete exposure of the lateral aspect of the tibia. A modification of the anteromedial approach has been recently described by Assal and colleagues[34] and allows excellent visualization of the anterior, anterolateral, and medial aspects of the articular and metaphyseal areas of the distal tibia, including the medial malleolus. The main disadvantage to this approach is the reliance on the often-tenuous soft tissue envelope of the distal anteromedial tibial surface.

The skin incision for the modified anteromedial approach begins longitudinally approximately 1–2 cm lateral to the anterior crest of the tibia and over the anterior compartment. This longitudinal component is continued distally to the level of the ankle joint at which point the incision curves medially to create an angle between the vertical and the horizontal limbs of approximately 105–110°. The horizontal incision extends to a point approximately 1 cm distal to the tip of the medial malleolus but frequently terminates once the saphenous vein is identified. A full thickness skin and subcutaneous tissue flap is elevated approximately 1–2 cm medially until the medial edge of the tibialis anterior tendon is identified. The tibial anterior tendon is protected and the extensor retinaculum and periosteum immediately medial to the tibialis tendon sheath is incised sharply. A full thickness skin, subcutaneous, and periosteal tissue flap is then elevated from the distal tibial metaphyseal region. Elevation of the anterior compartment with lateral retraction allows access to the lateral aspect of the distal tibia. A longitudinal capsulotomy is performed at the main fracture separation between the medial aspect of the Chaput fragment and the lateral aspect of the medial malleolar fragment. The capsulotomy should be carried onto the talar neck to allow adequate visualization. A universal distractor is applied using Schanz pins placed bicortically through the anteromedial surface of the tibial diaphysis and through the talar neck. The 4-mm talar neck pin is placed through the horizontal limb of the approach and under direct visualization (**Fig. 5**). This pin is placed transversely and in an extra-articular

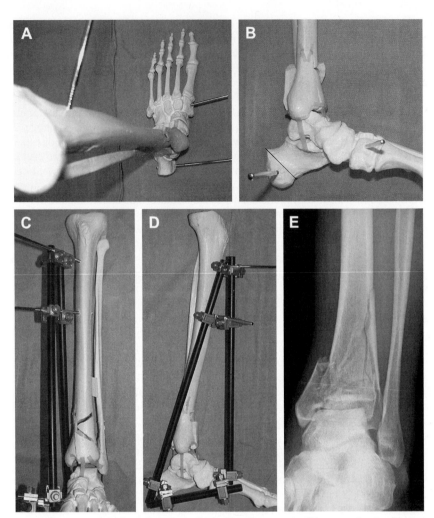

Fig. 1. Sawbones model of a left C-type tibial pilon fracture. In this example, the fibula has already been stabilized. (*A*) Medial aspect of the lower leg viewed from superiorly, demonstrating the orientation of pin placement in the proximal tibia, calcaneus, and midfoot (cuneiform). (*B*) The medial aspect of the foot demonstrating appropriate placement of the calcaneal and cuneiform pins. To minimize injury to the medial calcaneal neurovascular structures, the calcaneal pin should be placed posterior to the solid black line. The final reduction and appearance of the temporary medial spanning external fixator as viewed from the anterior (*C*) and lateral (*D*) viewpoints. An additional tibial pin has been inserted. Note that the tibial pins have been placed well proximal, to avoid anticipated skin incisions or implants. Anteroposterior (AP) (*E*) and lateral (*F*) plain radiographs of a C-type left tibial pilon fracture. The fibula is intact. Note the marked proximal and anterior translation of the talus. Anteroposterior (*G*) and lateral (*H*) plain radiographs after closed manipulative reduction and application of a medially-based external fixator. Substantial improvement in length, rotation, and alignment has been achieved.

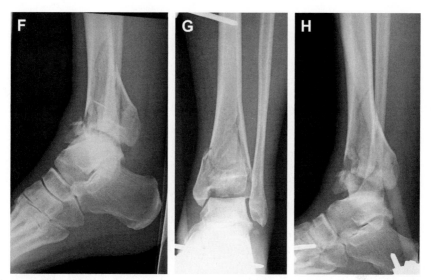

Fig. 1. (*continued*)

fashion. Occasionally, distraction preferentially occurs through the medial malleolar fragment (via traction through the deltoid ligament) or a comminuted metaphysis rather than through the tibiotalar articulation. In these situations, provisional stabilization of the medial malleolus and/or metaphysis may be required to allow joint distraction to occur. Through this approach, stabilizing implants can be placed directly onto the medial and anterolateral aspects of the distal tibia. If needed, the proximal portion(s) of the plate(s) and screws can be placed submuscularly or subcutaneously.

Wound closure is performed in layers. The capsule is repaired using absorbable sutures. The periosteal and retinacular flap is closed with an absorbable figure-eight suture technique. Importantly, each suture is placed and held with a hemostat clamp. After all of these deep sutures have been placed, an assistant applies traction to the hemostats to effect a reapproximation of the periosteal and retinacular interval while the surgeon definitively ties the sutures sequentially. A secure deep closure greatly decreases the amount of tension required to close the skin. A drain is placed beneath the subcutaneous flap. No subcutaneous sutures are required. An Allgower-Donati suture[21] is used to close skin with the knots tied at the lateral and distal aspect of the surgical incision.

Anterolateral approach The anterolateral approach avoids dissection over the tenuous soft tissue envelope of the distal tibia and is an excellent alternative to the anteromedial exposures. Visualization of medial shoulder comminution is more difficult than with the modified anteromedial approach, but the anterolateral approach otherwise allows excellent access to the vast majority of the tibial plafond. The exposure exploits the fracture involving the Chaput fragment, which is manipulated and typically externally rotated on the anterior tibiofibular ligament to allow access to the posterior and central aspects of the plafond. Anterolateral plate application is simplified with this exposure because the contents of the anterior compartment are retracted medially. If needed, medial implants can be placed percutaneously or through a separate medial malleolar approach (**Fig. 6**). The anterolateral approach for the distal tibia is an extension of the Bohler approach, which was previously described for operative fixation of talar neck fractures.[35]

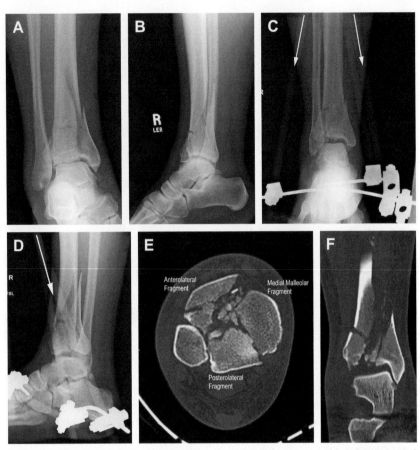

Fig. 2. Injury mortise (*A*) and lateral (*B*) plain radiographs of a 34 year-old male taken 12 days after falling 12 ft from a ladder. Because of his late presentation, displacement, and soft tissue swelling, the patient was initially treated with spanning external fixation using a delta-frame configuration (*C* and *D*). The force vectors to maintain the reduction are indicated by the white arrows, and parallel the orientation of the longitudinally oriented external fixation bars. Axial (*E*), coronal (*F*), and sagittal (*G*) computerized tomographic scanning after spanning external fixation demonstrates three major articular components: a medial malleolar fragment, an anterolateral (Chaput) fragment, and a posterior malleolar (Volkmann) fragment. Articular comminution is noted between all fracture fragments, most notably at the central intersection of all three fragments. After soft tissue recovery occurred, definitive ORIF was performed using an anteromedial surgical exposure. Intraoperative fluoroscopic images demonstrate satisfactory provisional reduction maintained with a bone holding clamp and multiple K-wires on the mortise (*H*) and lateral (*I*) views. Care is taken to ensure that the provisional fixation devices do not interfere with the definitive implants. An under-contoured malleable T-plate is applied to the anterior aspect of the distal tibia to secure the anterolateral and posterolateral articular fragments (*J*). Multiple screw fixations are inserted to definitively secure the majority of the articular portion of the tibial plafond (*K*). Final mortise (*L*) and lateral (*M*) immediate postoperative radiographs demonstrate a satisfactory articular reduction and restoration of distal tibial alignment. Because of the inherent tendency for this injury pattern to redisplace into varus malalignment, an additional stiff medial implant was applied.

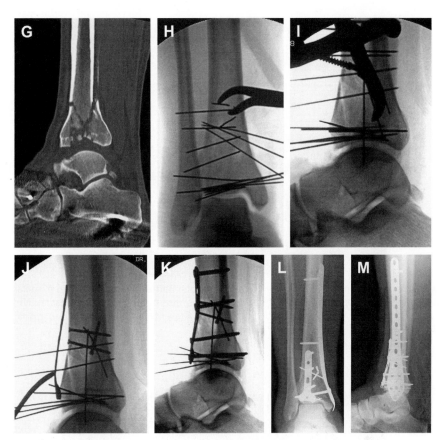

Fig. 2. (*continued*)

The skin incision is oriented longitudinally and in line with the fourth ray. Immediately within the subcutaneous fat, the superficial peroneal nerve and/or its arborizations are identified. The nerve and its branches are mobilized to allow retraction either medially or laterally. The distal extent of the fascia overlying the anterior compartment and its confluence with the extensor retinaculum are identified. With close observation, the tendons of the anterior compartment musculature can be identified. The extensor retinaculum is then incised longitudinally immediately lateral to the course of the long toe extensor tendons and peroneus tertius. The entire contents of the anterior compartment are then retracted medially to expose the underlying anterolateral aspect of the distal tibia and the capsule of the ankle joint. Care is taken when inserting the retractors below the anterior compartment as the anterior neurovascular bundle (anterior tibial artery and vein, and deep peroneal nerve) may be entrapped within anterior fracture fragments or, after 1–2 weeks from the time of injury, adherent to the this region. A longitudinal capsulotomy is performed at the medial extent of the Chaput fragment thereby exposing the tibiotalar articulation. A laterally-based Universal distractor is applied using Schanz pins placed from lateral to medial through the tibial diaphysis and from lateral to medial through the talar neck (**Fig. 7**). The central and posterior aspects of the tibial plafond are accessed by externally rotating the anterolateral (Chaput) fragment on the anterior distal tibiofibular syndesmotic ligaments.

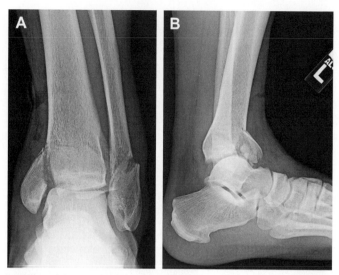

Fig. 3. Mortise (*A*) and lateral (*B*) plain radiographs of a partial articular injury. In this example, the posterior aspect of the tibial plafond remains in continuity with the metadiaphyseal portion of the tibia. Substantial comminution of the anterior aspect of the plafond is identified.

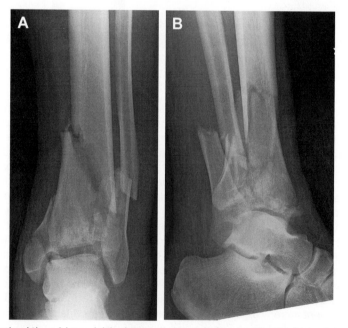

Fig. 4. Mortise (*A*) and lateral (*B*) plain radiographs of a complete articular injury. In this example, the entirety of the articular surface of the tibial plafond is separate from the distal metadiaphysis of the tibia. Significant comminution of the articular surface can be identified.

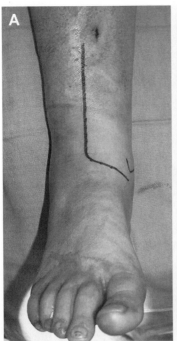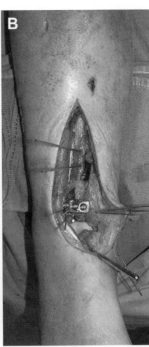

Fig. 5. (A) The proposed surgical incision has been marked out on this patient's right ankle. Note that the vertical component of the incision is immediately lateral to the palpable anterior tibial crest. After the ankle joint is passed, the incision curves to a point approximately 1 cm distal to the tip of the medial malleolus. (B) Deep surgical exposure demonstrating the transition from provisional to definitive fixation for a displaced tibial pilon fracture using the modified anteromedial exposure. Notice that the tibialis anterior tendon and the entirety of the anterior compartment are retracted laterally.

Posterolateral approach The posterolateral approach is an extremely useful exposure to access and manipulate the posterior aspect of the tibial plafond.[17,18] It is most useful for those B-type tibial pilon fractures where the unstable articular segment is located posteriorly and has no significant articular comminution. Although the posterolateral approach is uncommonly used in isolation for the management of C-type tibial pilon fractures, it can be used in conjunction with anterior exposures to adequately reduce and stabilize the entire articular surface. C-type fracture patterns most amenable to this adjunctive approach include: those with complete dissociation of the Volkmann fragment from the fibula, especially those that remain substantially displaced despite anatomic reduction of any associated fibula fracture; and those articular injury patterns that demonstrate a large minimally comminuted posterior plafond fragment that can be anatomically reduced to the posterior metadiaphysis effectively converting a C-type tibial pilon fracture into a B-type pattern.[12] Direct visualization of the articular surface is extremely difficult, if not impossible, with this exposure. The articular reduction is largely indirect, is accomplished based on a visual inspection of any available posterior cortical interdigitations, and is confirmed radiographically. Fibular fixation using this same skin incision is also possible but requires posterior retraction of the peroneal musculature. Because this exposure can be performed in conjunction with operative fixation of the fibula, it is imperative that the surgeon considers all the anticipated skin incisions required when proceeding with any

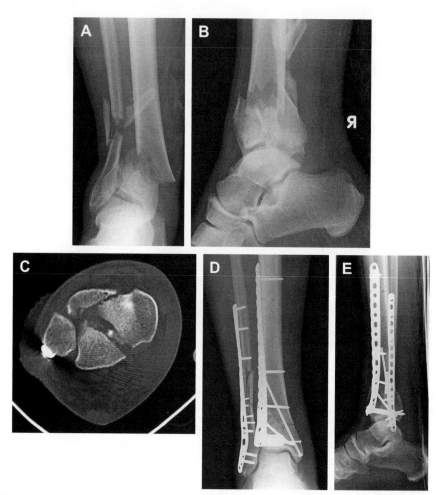

Fig. 6. Injury anteroposterior (A) and lateral (B) plain radiographs of a displaced right tibial pilon fracture that occurred during a motorcycle accident. The distal tibial soft tissues demonstrated substantial swelling with severe contusion of the medial skin. Initial management included open reduction and internal fixation (ORIF) of the comminuted fibula fracture and application of a medial spanning external fixator. Axial CT scanning demonstrated a relatively simple articular injury (C). Note the relatively large medial malleolar fragment with comminution identified centrally, between the medial malleolus and the posterolateral (Volkmann) fragment. Definitive ORIF was performed using an anterolateral surgical exposure after resolution of soft tissue swelling occurred. Immediate postoperative anteroposterior (D) and lateral (E) plain radiographs demonstrate satisfactory restoration of the articular surface and metadiaphyseal alignment.

surgical management of these fractures. For example, a poorly positioned fibular incision may substantially jeopardize the ability to use the posterolateral exposure.

To facilitate the posterolateral exposure, the patient is positioned either laterally or prone. The skin incision is longitudinally oriented midway between the lateral aspect of the Achilles tendon and the posterolateral aspect of the fibula. Care is taken to avoid injury to the sural nerve. The deep fascia is incised and the peroneal musculature is identified and retracted laterally. The surgeon then works posterior to the fibula and

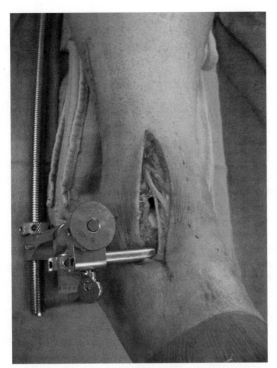

Fig. 7. Intraoperative photograph of the right lower leg viewed from the anterolateral aspect. An anterolateral surgical exposure has been performed and a universal distractor has been applied; the Schanz pin has been inserted from lateral to medial through the talar neck. Note the arborizing superficial peroneal nerve centrally located within the exposure.

identifies the fascia covering the flexor hallucis longus muscle. The flexor hallucis longus musculature is then elevated from lateral to medial from the posterior aspect of the tibia. The posterolateral aspect of the distal tibia is subsequently identified.

Posteromedial approach The posteromedial approach is uncommonly required for the management of tibial pilon fractures. Occasional indications include posterior pilon variant fractures with substantial central and/or posterior comminution with an intact anterior plafond, or the tibial pilon fracture with an associated large posteromedial fragment that can be accessed and secured at its metadiaphyseal junction.[12]

The posteromedial approach can be accomplished with the patient positioned supine or prone. If the patient is in the supine position, a bump is placed under the contralateral buttock and flank region thereby facilitating external rotation of the injured leg. Occasionally, the prone position is used and allows an easier trajectory for the insertion of screws and provisional stabilizing wires. The incision is typically halfway between the medial border of the Achilles tendon and the posterior aspect of the medial malleolus. After the tarsal tunnel is entered, the neurovascular bundle is identified and protected. The specific deep interval depends on the fracture type and the access needed. However, after the neurovascular bundle is mobilized, dissection can proceed through any interval within the tarsal tunnel.

Reduction and fixation sequence
The reduction and fixation sequence of any tibial pilon fracture varies according to the specific fracture anatomy, condition of the local soft tissues, and technical ability and

experience of the surgeon. Reduction of the articular portion of a tibial pilon injury remains the most critical aspect of surgical care and, therefore, typically dominates the surgical tactic, reduction sequence, choice of exposure(s), and application of stabilizing implants. Invariably, the posterolateral fragment is critically assessed as the starting point for the majority of C-type fracture patterns. Reduction of this Volkmann's fragment is frequently accomplished with anatomic reduction and stabilization of the fibula fracture. If satisfactorily reduced, the reduction sequence typically involves reducing the posterior aspect of the medial malleolar fragment to the Volkmann fragment. Central comminution is then disimpacted and reduced to the posterior plafond. Bone graft material can be used to maintain the reduction of this associated impaction. The medial malleolar fragment is secured using the medial shoulder chondral interdigitations, followed by reduction of the anterolateral (Chaput) fragment. Provisional fixation is accomplished with the use of strategically applied clamps and Kirschner wires (K-wires). Occasionally, the posterolateral plafond demonstrates a dorsiflexion impaction injury that can be appreciated by critically assessing the sagittal CT reformations. In this situation, subsequent reductions to the posterior plafond result in an extension deformity of the articular surface and altered contact pressures affecting the anterior plafond. It is imperative that the surgeon identifies this posterolateral impaction injury and rotates the affected plafond segment into a reduced position before proceeding with the remaining reduction maneuvers.

One of the most useful strategies for reduction of the articular segment as well as reduction of the metadiaphysis is to identify a fracture fragment that contains a reasonable amount of articular surface distally and a minimally comminuted metaphyseal or metadiaphyseal proximal extension. In this situation, anatomic reduction of the proximal metadiaphyseal component essentially converts the C-type tibial pilon fracture into a partial articular (B-type) injury, greatly facilitating the reduction of the remaining articular surface and providing a basis for reduction of axial alignment. Large medial malleolar fragments, posterior osteochondral fragments, or large Volkmann fragments are typically those that are sought for this reduction strategy.

Provisional stabilizing implants are critical for the success of the procedure. Invariably, these temporizing implants include numerous small diameter K-wires, strategically placed clamps, and minifragment plates and screws. These devices should be placed out of the zone of definitive implants and therefore a pre-existing knowledge of the definitive implants, reduction sequence, and choices of surgical approaches is mandatory.

Definitive internal fixation

Historically, implants used for stabilization of tibial pilon fractures were placed on the anteromedial surface of the tibia. The usefulness of these implants was limited by their bulkiness, nonanatomic design, and limited areas for strategic screw placement. Contemporary implants use a lower profile with more anatomically-based design, allowing percutaneous and plate reduction techniques. The goals of definitive internal fixation should include absolute stability and interfragmentary compression of reduced articular segments, stable fixation of the articular segment to the tibial diaphysis, and restoration of coronal, transverse, and sagittal plane alignments. The location, rigidity, and number of these implants are based on each individual fracture. Factors to consider include: the degree of comminution; the ability to achieve cortical contact and intrinsic fracture stability; the bone quality; the direction of the initial failure of the bone (varus, valgus, flexion, extension); the status of the soft tissue envelope; and any associated bone loss, among others.[13] It is important to recognize that the majority of implant placements onto the proximal intact segment of the tibia can be performed indirectly, using a submuscular plate insertion along the anterolateral aspect of the tibia through the anterolateral approach, and by using a percutaneous medial plate placement. Invariably, the plate thickness should balance the need for an implant that has adequate stiffness to counter the anticipated loads, while maintaining a minimum amount of plate prominence and injury to the soft tissue envelope particularly along the anteromedial surface of the tibia. When neutralizing C-type injuries, at least one stiff (eg, 3.5-mm compression plate) implant is usually required to maintain metadiaphyseal alignment (See **Fig. 2**). B-type injuries do not require metadiaphyseal neutralization and they can commonly be managed with lower profile implants that allow effective neutralization of the reduced partial articular injury.

Locked plating remains poorly defined for intra-articular fractures of the distal tibia, and current evidence-based recommendations are lacking. Relative indications include poor bone quality, anticipated prolonged time to union (particularly in those with metaphyseal bone loss), or situations where the ideal choice of implants cannot be performed secondary to local soft tissue conditions. The majority of tibial pilon fractures at the authors' institution continue to be managed with nonlocking screw-plate devices.

Rehabilitation

At the conclusion of the surgical procedure, patients are placed into a well-padded plaster splint with the foot in neutral position. The wound is typically examined in the outpatient clinic area approximately 4–5 days later. Splinting with the foot in neutral is continued until the sutures are removed at the 2–3 week mark. A supervised physical therapy program consisting of active, active-assisted, and passive range of motion of the ankle, subtalar, and metatarsophalangeal joints is subsequently initiated. To avoid equinus contracture, a removable nighttime and resting splint is recommended. Weight-bearing is typically delayed for approximately 12 weeks, at which point the patient begins partial progressive weight-bearing in a removable boot. The physical therapy focus at this point consists of maximization of motion, strengthening, gait training, and the weaning of ambulatory devices such as crutches, canes, and external supports. Postoperatively, edema may be substantial and persist for several months following injury. In addition to patient education regarding this normal phenomenon, an elastic stocking is provided to help decrease dependency-related swelling.

The Nonreconstructable Pilon

At the authors' institution, all efforts at restoring normal anatomy are performed. However, tibial pilon fractures may present with such significant comminution, bone loss, soft tissue injury, or associated patient factors that the risks of ORIF are far in excess of any potential benefit. These are unique situations and multiple opinions regarding the best form of functional salvage should be sought.

Patients presenting with an acute overt loss of a substantial amount of osteoarticular bone in the context of an open fracture may be best served with a staged tibiotalar arthrodesis. In the younger patient with this injury pattern, staged osteoarticular allograft reconstruction may be reasonable, however, long-term results of most osteoarticular allografts performed for joint reconstructions after tumor resecting procedures demonstrate limited longevity of the allograft. This type of osteochondral bone loss should be differentiated from those patients with open fractures who present with nonarticular supramalleolar bone loss. In these latter patients, an attempt at limb salvage using staged articular and axial reduction and stabilization, followed by soft tissue transfer if needed, and delayed bone grafting have demonstrated satisfactory results at achieving union with an acceptable complication rate.[36] Patients presenting with closed fractures but articular comminution that is so severe that restoration of articular congruity is felt to be futile are unusual. In these situations, the articular surface is ignored and the treatment goals are as follows: restoration of axial alignment such that the talus is centered beneath the long axis of the tibia in the coronal and sagittal planes, obtaining metadiaphyseal union, and choosing a stabilizing technique that does not compromise later tibiotalar arthrodesis. In these unusual situations, these goals can be achieved with the use of an ankle spanning external fixator or percutaneous plating. In rare situations, particularly in low demand individuals with severe injuries, hindfoot fusion nailing can be performed acutely, understanding that the goals are to provide a plantigrade, comfortable foot with minimization of wound complications and complex surgical procedures.

Rarely, the authors have performed an accurate acute articular reduction with screw fixation followed by transarticular spanning external fixation. In these situations, the strategy includes staged nonunion repair of the metadiaphysis if the patient recovers from their other injuries or illnesses and the local soft tissue envelope is amenable to reconstruction. In some situations, however, a well-timed below-the-knee amputation remains one of the most functional procedures available for the nonreconstructable tibial pilon fracture and it should be considered as an option alongside those listed in all of the preceding scenarios.

OUTCOMES

Although the outcomes of tibial pilon fractures are affected by numerous variables including the osteochondral injury and treatment method chosen, perhaps no factor is as important as the degree of initial soft tissue injury.[29] The initial enthusiasm for ORIF of tibial pilon fractures followed the successful reports by Ruedi.[1,7,37] When applied to the North American population, however, the associated soft tissue complications after ORIF were disastrous, with frequent soft tissue complications including deep infection.[8,9,22,29] Despite the recognition of an increased proportion of axial loading injuries in the North American population compared with the higher proportion of torsional injuries treated in the Ruedi study, the initial enthusiasm for ORIF waned and other treatment options were sought.

Treatment with external fixation emerged as the potential solution, and it was associated with a smaller surgical insult to the traumatized local soft tissues. This method of treatment, combined with an understanding of the impact of any soft tissue insult on potential complications, contributed to a satisfactory outcome in some patients.[23,25,27-29,38-42] However, problems with maintenance of axial alignment and difficulties with residual articular incongruity became evident. As the appreciation for the soft tissue envelope evolved, a two-staged protocol was initiated that consists of an initial period of restoring length, alignment, rotation, and stability to the injured limb via the use of ORIF of any associated fibula fracture, and the application of a temporary ankle joint spanning external fixator.[10,11] Definitive ORIF of the tibia was then performed after resolution of soft tissue edema and blisters occurred. Currently, this staged protocol has demonstrated its effectiveness in substantially decreasing soft tissue complications compared with the initial North American experience.

Long-term results of tibial pilon fractures demonstrate a significant impact on physical function despite satisfactory initial reductions. Pollak and colleagues noted that at a minimum of 2 years from injury, patients still demonstrated significant pain, swelling, and disability with both ORIF and external fixation.[43] Interesting, external fixation was identified as the only surgeon-controlled variable associated with poorer outcome measures. Marsh similarly identified substantial impairment in tibial pilon fractures at 5 years using external fixation and percutaneous screw treatments.[44]

In summary, the recognition of the soft tissue injury has evolved as a critical component of the management of these injuries. Circular external fixation, staged protocols for ORIF, and limited exposures with percutaneous techniques have all contributed to a decreased incidence of deep wound complications compared with those in the early 1970s. Long-term functional outcomes, however, remain poor secondary to residual pain and disability from ankle stiffness, arthritis, prolonged time to function, and the number of surgical procedures. Despite these later problems, the surgical approach currently entails recognition of the soft tissue injury, a staged approach to allow resolution of edema before proceeding, and definitive fixation with accurate articular reduction and axial alignment.

SUMMARY

High-energy fractures of the tibial plafond are a life-changing event for the patient. Currently, open reduction and internal fixation appears to offer the best chance for obtaining and maintaining anatomic articular reduction and axial alignment to union. Definitive ORIF should be performed in a staged fashion to allow adequate resolution of the associated soft tissue injury. A preoperative plan is essential to a successful outcome and it must include a strategy to access and stabilize the articular and nonarticular components of the injury.

REFERENCES

1. Ruedi T, Matter P, Allgower M. Die intraartikullaeren Frakturen des distalen Unterschenkelendes. Helv Chir Acta 1968;35(5):556–82.
2. Kellam JF, Waddell JP. Fractures of the distal tibial metaphysis with intra-articular extension–the distal tibial explosion fracture. J Trauma 1979;19(8):593–601.
3. Bourne RB, Rorabeck CH, Macnab J. Intra-articular fractures of the distal tibia: the pilon fracture. J Trauma 1983;23(7):591–6.
4. Ovadia DN, Beals RK. Fractures of the tibial plafond. J Bone Joint Surg Am 1986; 68(4):543–51.
5. Tornetta P III, Gorup J. Axial computed tomography of pilon fractures. Clin Orthop Relat Res 1996 Feb;(323):273–6.
6. Ruedi T, Allgower M. Spatresultate nach operativer Behandlung der Gelenkbruche am distalen Tibiaende (sog. Pilon-Frakturen). Unfallheilkunde 1978; 81(4):319–23.
7. Ruedi TP, Allgower M. The operative treatment of intra-articular fractures of the lower end of the tibia. Clin Orthop Relat Res 1979 Jan-Feb;(138):105–10.
8. McFerran MA, Smith SW, Boulas HJ, et al. Complications encountered in the treatment of pilon fractures. J Orthop Trauma 1992;6(2):195–200.
9. Teeny SM, Wiss DA. Open reduction and internal fixation of tibial plafond fractures. Variables contributing to poor results and complications. Clin Orthop Relat Res 1993 Jul;(292):108–17.
10. Patterson MJ, Cole JD. Two-staged delayed open reduction and internal fixation of severe pilon fractures. J Orthop Trauma 1999;13(2):85–91.
11. Sirkin M, Sanders R, DiPasquale T, et al. A staged protocol for soft tissue management in the treatment of complex pilon fractures. J Orthop Trauma 1999;13(2):78–84.

12. Dunbar RP, Barei DP, Kubiak EN, et al. Early limited internal fixation of diaphyseal extensions in select pilon fractures: upgrading AO/OTA type C fractures to AO/OTA type B. J Orthop Trauma 2008;22(6):426–9.

13. Nork SE. Distal tibia fractures. In: Stannard JP, Schmidt AH, Kregor PJ, editors. Surgical treatment of orthopaedic trauma. New York: Thieme; 2007. p. 767–91.

14. Wissing JC, van Laarhoven CJ, van der Werken C. The posterior antiglide plate for fixation of fractures of the lateral malleolus. Injury 1992;23(2):94–6.

15. Ostrum RF. Posterior plating of displaced Weber B fibula fractures. J Orthop Trauma 1996;10(3):199–203.

16. Howard JL, Agel J, Barei DP, et al. A prospective study evaluating incision placement and wound healing for tibial plafond fractures. J Orthop Trauma 2008;22(5):299–305 [discussion: 6].

17. Konrath GA, Hopkins G II. Posterolateral approach for tibial pilon fractures: a report of two cases. J Orthop Trauma 1999;13(8):586–9.

18. Bhattacharyya T, Crichlow R, Gobezie R, et al. Complications associated with the posterolateral approach for pilon fractures. J Orthop Trauma 2006;20(2):104–7.

19. Casey D, McConnell T, Parekh S, et al. Percutaneous pin placement in the medial calcaneus: is anywhere safe? J Orthop Trauma 2002;16(1):26–9.

20. Weber BG. Lengthening osteotomy of the fibula to correct a widened mortice of the ankle after fracture. Int Orthop 1981;4(4):289–93.

21. Sagi HC, Papp S, Dipasquale T. The effect of suture pattern and tension on cutaneous blood flow as assessed by laser Doppler flowmetry in a pig model. J Orthop Trauma 2008;22(3):171–5.

22. Wyrsch B, McFerran MA, McAndrew M, et al. Operative treatment of fractures of the tibial plafond. A randomized, prospective study. J Bone Joint Surg Am 1996; 78(11):1646–57.

23. Anglen JO. Early outcome of hybrid external fixation for fracture of the distal tibia. J Orthop Trauma 1999;13(2):92–7.

24. Blauth M, Bastian L, Krettek C, et al. Surgical options for the treatment of severe tibial pilon fractures: a study of three techniques. J Orthop Trauma 2001;15(3): 153–60.

25. Bonar SK, Marsh JL. Unilateral external fixation for severe pilon fractures. Foot Ankle 1993;14(2):57–64.

26. Barbieri R, Schenk R, Koval K, et al. Hybrid external fixation in the treatment of tibial plafond fractures. Clin Orthop Relat Res 1996 Nov;(332):16–22.

27. Court-Brown CM, Walker C, Garg A, et al. Half-ring external fixation in the management of tibial plafond fractures. J Orthop Trauma 1999;13(3):200–6.

28. French B, Tornetta P III. Hybrid external fixation of tibial pilon fractures. Foot Ankle Clin 2000;5(4):853–71.

29. Watson JT, Moed BR, Karges DE, et al. Pilon fractures. Treatment protocol based on severity of soft tissue injury. Clin Orthop Relat Res 2000 Jun;(375):78–90.

30. Etter C, Ganz R. Long-term results of tibial plafond fractures treated with open reduction and internal fixation. Arch Orthop Trauma Surg 1991;110(6):277–83.

31. Marsh JL, Buckwalter J, Gelberman R, et al. Articular fractures: does an anatomic reduction really change the result? J Bone Joint Surg Am 2002;84(7): 1259–71.

32. Topliss CJ, Jackson M, Atkins RM. Anatomy of pilon fractures of the distal tibia. J Bone Joint Surg Br 2005;87(5):692–7.

33. Sommer C, Ruedi T. Tibia: distal (pilon). In: Ruedi TP, Murphy WM, editors. AO principles of fracture management. Stuttgart: Thieme; 2000. p. 539–57.

34. Assal M, Ray A, Stern R. The extensile approach for the operative treatment of high-energy pilon fractures: surgical technique and soft-tissue healing. J Orthop Trauma 2007;21(3):198–206.

35. Herscovici D Jr, Sanders RW, Infante A, et al. Bohler incision: an extensile anterolateral approach to the foot and ankle. J Orthop Trauma 2000;14(6): 429–32.

36. Gardner MJ, Mehta S, Barei DP, et al. Treatment protocol for open AO/OTA type C3 pilon fractures with segmental bone loss. J Orthop Trauma 2008;22(7):451–7.

37. Ruedi T. Fractures of the lower end of the tibia into the ankle joint: results 9 years after open reduction and internal fixation. Injury 1973;5(2):130–4.

38. Murphy CP, D'Ambrosia R, Dabezies EJ. The small pin circular fixator for distal tibial pilon fractures with soft tissue compromise. Orthopedics 1991;14(3): 283–90.

39. Bone L, Stegemann P, McNamara K, et al. External fixation of severely comminuted and open tibial pilon fractures. Clin Orthop Relat Res 1993 Jul;(292):101–7.

40. Tornetta P III, Weiner L, Bergman M, et al. Pilon fractures: treatment with combined internal and external fixation. J Orthop Trauma 1993;7(6):489–96.

41. Bonar SK, Marsh JL. Tibial plafond fractures: changing principles of treatment. J Am Acad Orthop Surg 1994;2(6):297–305.

42. Marsh JL, Bonar S, Nepola JV, et al. Use of an articulated external fixator for fractures of the tibial plafond. J Bone Joint Surg Am 1995;77(10):1498–509.

43. Pollak AN, McCarthy ML, Bess RS, et al. Outcomes after treatment of high-energy tibial plafond fractures. J Bone Joint Surg Am 2003;85(10):1893–900.

44. Marsh JL, Weigel DP, Dirschl DR. Tibial plafond fractures. How do these ankles function over time? J Bone Joint Surg Am 2003;85(2):287–95.

A Rational Approach to Ankle Fractures

Michael P. Clare, MD

KEYWORDS

• Ankle • Malleolus • Fracture • Treatment

Ankle fractures are among the most common of all fractures, and the ankle joint represents the most commonly injured weight-bearing joint.[1] Compared with pilon fractures, ankle fractures are typically the result of lower energy, rotational injury mechanisms. which have a lower inherent incidence of post-traumatic arthritis. However, ankle fractures represent a spectrum of injury patterns from simple to complex, such that these injuries are not always "just an ankle fracture." What follows is an attempt to outline a rational approach to the management of ankle fractures.

BIOMECHANICAL CONSIDERATIONS

The ankle joint is subject to enormous forces across a relatively small surface area of contact, with up to 1.5 times body weight with gait and greater than 5.5 times body weight with more strenuous activity. Maintaining congruency of the ankle joint is therefore critical to the long-term viability of the ankle. Ramsey and Hamilton[2] showed in a cadaveric model that only 1 mm of lateral translation of the talus reduced surface contact area in the ankle joint by 42%; lateral translation of 2mm reduced surface contact area in the ankle joint by 64%. Decreased surface contact area leads to an abnormal distribution of joint stresses, which presumably leads to post-traumatic arthritis.[2] Similarly, Thordarson and colleagues[3] showed that 2 mm of shortening or lateral shift of the fibula, or external rotation greater than or equal to 5 degrees, increases contact forces in the ankle joint, which may predispose to ankle arthritis.

Mechanically, the fibula functions as a post to resist lateral translation of the talus. The posterior malleolus acts as a restraint against posterior translation of the talus, and fractures involving approximately 25% of the articular surface will result in posterior instability. The medial malleolus includes the anterior colliculus, onto which the superficial deltoid ligament attaches, and the posterior colliculus, which anchors the deep deltoid ligament. The deep deltoid ligament is a primary static stabilizer of the ankle joint and resists external rotation of the talus.

Florida Orthopaedic Institute, 13020 Telecom Parkway North Tampa, FL 33637, USA
E-mail address: mpclare@verizon.net

Foot Ankle Clin N Am 13 (2008) 593–610
doi:10.1016/j.fcl.2008.09.003
1083-7515/08/$ – see front matter © 2008 Elsevier Inc. All rights reserved.

foot.theclinics.com

CLASSIFICATION

The Lauge-Hansen classification was developed in 1950 as a result of both cadaveric dissections of experimentally produced fractures, and clinical and radiographic examinations.[4] Four consistent patterns were recognized: supination-external rotation, supination-adduction, pronation-abduction, and pronation-external rotation. The work was a landmark advance because it was the first classification scheme to assign a causative mechanism of injury to ankle fractures that, with the subsequent development of arbeitsgemeinschaft für osteosynthesefragen (A-O) principles of internal fixation, provided guidance for treatment.

Each of the four patterns is subdivided into stages that can be used to determine the inherent stability of the injury. The classification involves a two-term nomenclature: the first term describes the position of the foot, and the second term describes the direction of force applied. With supination, the lateral structures are on tension; with pronation, the medial structures are on tension.

INJURY PATTERNS
Supination-External Rotation

The supination-external rotation (S-ER) pattern is the most common injury pattern and accounts for 40%–75% of all ankle fractures. A supination-external rotation injury includes: (I) failure of the anterior-inferior tibiofibular ligament (AITFL); (II) a spiral oblique fibula fracture at or just above the ankle mortise; (III) failure of the posterior-inferior tibiofibular ligament (PITFL) or posterior malleolus fracture; and (IV) tension failure of the deep deltoid ligament or transverse avulsion fracture of the medial malleolus (**Fig. 1**). Tornetta described the combination medial injury variant, which includes tension failure of the deep deltoid ligament and an avulsion fracture of the anterior colliculus (**Fig. 2**).[5]

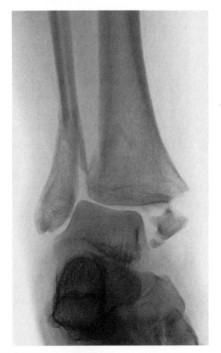

Fig. 1. Supination–external rotation pattern.

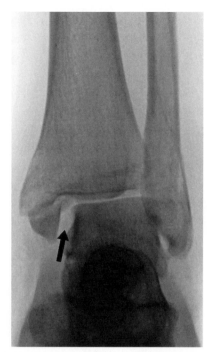

Fig. 2. Combination medial injury. Note widening of medial clear space (*arrow*) and medial malleolar fracture.

Supination-Adduction

The supination-adduction (S-AD) pattern accounts for 10%–20% of ankle fractures. A supination-adduction pattern includes: (I) a low avulsion fracture of the lateral malleolus or lateral ligament injury; and (II) a vertical shear fracture of the medial malleolus (**Fig. 3**). This pattern is also associated with an impaction injury to the medial tibial plafond.[6]

Pronation-Abduction

The pronation-abduction (P-AB) pattern accounts for 5%–20% of ankle fractures and is commonly associated with instability of the syndesmosis. A pronation-abduction pattern includes: (I) tension failure of the deep deltoid ligament or transverse avulsion fracture of the medial malleolus; (II) failure of the AITFL and PITFL; and (III) a transverse fibula fracture at or above the ankle mortise, typically with lateral comminution because of the bending forces applied to the fibula (**Fig. 4**). This pattern is also associated with an impaction injury to the lateral tibial plafond.

Pronation-External Rotation

The pronation-external rotation (P-ER) pattern accounts for 7%–19% of ankle fractures and includes the Maisonneuve injury. A pronation-external rotation pattern includes: (I) tension failure of the deep deltoid ligament or transverse avulsion fracture of the medial malleolus; (II) failure of the AITFL; (III) a spiral oblique fibula fracture above the ankle mortise; and (IV) failure of the PITFL or posterior malleolus fracture (**Fig. 5**). This pattern is also commonly associated with instability of the syndesmosis.

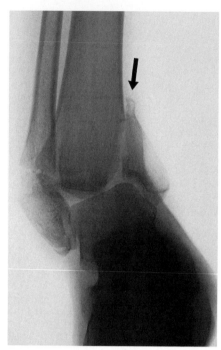

Fig. 3. Supination–adduction pattern. Note vertical orientation of medial fracture line (*arrow*).

RADIOGRAPHIC CONSIDERATIONS

Certain preliminary radiographic criteria are beneficial in determining the relative stability or instability of a malleolar fracture. Coronal plane symmetry, particularly in the absence of fracture medially, can be assessed with respect to the medial and lateral clear spaces. Preservation of fibular length and the so-called "Shenton's line of the ankle" imply some degree of inherent stability (**Fig. 6**). Sagittal plane symmetry can be assessed with respect to the presence or absence of a posterior malleolar fracture, which because of the PITFL attachment typically provides an indirect indication of fibular length.

DECISION-MAKING IN ANKLE FRACTURES

In the event of a suspected ankle fracture, clinical evaluation includes a thorough patient history as to the injury mechanism, and the anticipated force and energy involved. The reported injury mechanism and radiographic fracture pattern are then used to classify the injury by the Lauge-Hansen classification.[4] Stable injury patterns can be treated nonoperatively; unstable injury patterns are typically treated operatively.

Difficulty can be encountered in diagnosing deltoid incompetence, primarily in the context of distinguishing an S-ER II pattern from an S-ER IV pattern. Previous studies have shown that medial tenderness, swelling, and ecchymosis are poor predictors of deltoid incompetence.[7–9] In the absence of distinct radiographic widening of the medial space and asymmetry of the ankle mortise, stress radiographs can be beneficial. Michelson, and colleagues[10] described the gravity stress test, in which the lateral portion of the ankle is positioned down on the radiographic table, with the majority of the

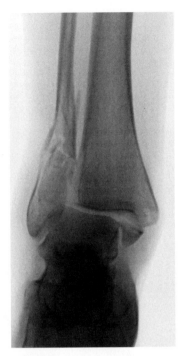

Fig. 4. Pronation–abduction pattern.

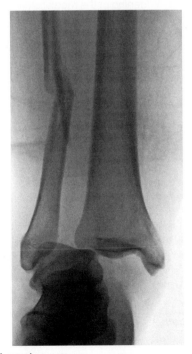

Fig. 5. Pronation–external rotation pattern.

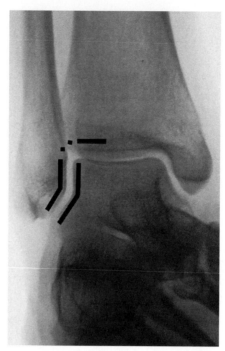

Fig. 6. Coronal plane symmetry. Note fibular length and symmetry through talofibular joint.

ankle off the edge of the table. Widening of the medial clear space on cross-table mortise radiograph is considered positive for deltoid incompetence. Others have advocated external rotation stress radiographs.[7–9] More recent studies have suggested that the gravity stress test is as reliable as the external rotation stress test and more comfortable for the patient.[11,12] Alternatively, the patient can be placed in a prefabricated fracture boot and allowed to weight-bear to tolerance; repeat weight-bearing radiographs are obtained 5–7 days later. Operative treatment is indicated in the event of subsequent medial clear space widening on follow-up radiographs.

OPERATIVE TREATMENT
General Considerations

In the absence of an open injury or irreducible dislocation, surgical treatment for an unstable ankle fracture pattern is certainly not an emergency and can therefore be completed as an elective procedure. The author prefers to delay definitive surgery for 10–14 days, until resolution of the acute inflammatory phase. This delay allows dissipation of soft tissue swelling, and in light of the limited soft tissue envelope surrounding the ankle joint, theoretically lessens the risk of wound complications. It also affords time for additional imaging studies, such as computed tomography (CT) scanning, when necessary, and completion of preoperative planning.

Principles of Internal Fixation

As with stabilization of any extremity fracture, strict adherence to A/O principles of internal fixation is of paramount importance in ensuring a favorable functional outcome.

These include: atraumatic soft tissue handling with minimal periosteal stripping; anatomic fracture reduction; (sufficiently) rigid internal fixation; and early range of motion.[13]

Fibular Length and Rotation

Restoration of fibular length and rotation is critical in reestablishing a stable ankle mortise, and can be assessed radiographically off of the talofibular articulation. In the instance of excessive comminution or poor bone quality, indirect reduction techniques can be beneficial in ensuring restoration of fibular length and rotation.[14] Using the indirect "push-pull" technique, the selected plate is initially secured to the distal fragment, and an additional screw is placed proximal to the plate, typically 4 mm longer than measured. An A/O laminar spreader is positioned between the supplemental screw and the proximal edge of the plate. As fibular length is restored under fluoroscopic guidance, the proximal fragment is provisionally secured to the plate with a small clamp **(Fig. 7)**.

OPERATIVE TREATMENT OF SPECIFIC INJURY PATTERNS
Supination-External Rotation

Fibular stabilization can be completed using either a dorsal anti-glide or lateral neutralization technique, typically with a simple one-third tubular plate and 3.5-mm cortical screws **(Fig. 8)**. Although there is no overall difference in fracture healing rates or overall outcome between the two fixation methods, the dorsal anti-glide plate offers several distinct advantages, including: less prominence and thus better soft tissue coverage and lower incidence of late hardware removal;[15–17] and a stronger overall construct.[18] Distal plate placement on the lateral malleolus or prominent distal screw heads is associated with a higher incidence of peroneal tendon irritation and tendinous lesions.[19]

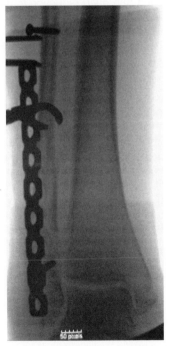

Fig. 7. Indirect push-pull technique. Note restoration of fibular length without disruption of fracture comminution.

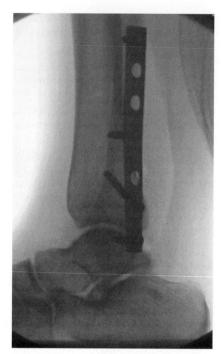

Fig. 8. Dorsal anti-glide fixation for supination–external rotation pattern.

Medially, the author prefers a true open reduction in which periosteum and other potential sources of soft tissue interposition, which may predispose the fracture to delayed union or nonunion, can be removed from within the fracture site. An open reduction additionally affords the opportunity for an arthrotomy through which the chondral surfaces can be assessed and loose bodies can be removed.

Supination-Adduction

There are multiple fixation options for the fibula, including: hook plate; single screw; or tension band constructs. The choice of fixation ultimately depends on the size of the fragment and amount of displacement: nondisplaced fractures can be stabilized by percutaneous retrograde screw fixation; the author prefers a hook plate for displaced fragments. Minimal avulsion fragments typically require no fixation.

Because of the vertical orientation of the fracture line, medial fixation must be positioned more transversely to prevent secondary shortening and displacement. The author prefers a 5-hole 1/3 tubular plate as an anti-glide or buttress device combined with lag screw fixation **(Fig. 9)**. The medial corner of the tibial plafond must also be assessed for impaction. In this instance, the fragment can be reflected distally to expose the impacted area. A small osteotome is used to gently disimpact the involved area, preserving the subchondral bone attached to the articular surface, and the cancellous defect is backfilled with bone graft substitute. The fragment is reduced and the area of impaction is supported with lag screw fixation directly above the fragment.

Pronation-Abduction

Because of the lateral comminution, bridge plate fixation is commonly required **(Fig. 10)**. In this instance, fibular length can be restored with the indirect push-pull

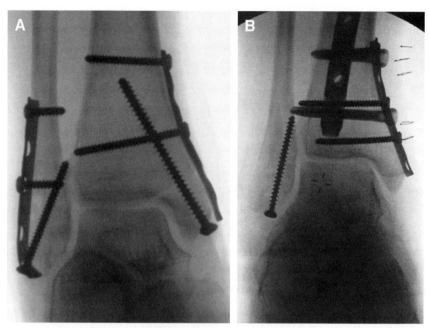

Fig. 9. Fixation of supination–adduction pattern: *A)* hook plate laterally and anti-glide fixation medially; *B)* single screw fixation laterally and anti-glide fixation medially.

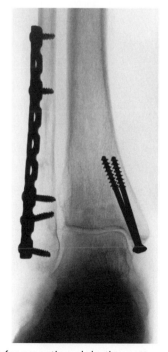

Fig. 10. Bridge plate fixation for pronation–abduction pattern.

technique described previously.[14] The author prefers a 3.5-mm reconstruction plate for these fractures; alternatively, this pattern may represent the lone indication in ankle fractures for a locking plate. Syndesmotic instability is anticipated, and stabilized where necessary. The lateral tibial plafond must also be assessed for impaction.

Pronation-External Rotation

Fibular fixation depends on how proximal the fracture extends. Fracture lines immediately proximal to the ankle mortise can be stabilized with a 1/3 tubular plate; more proximal fracture lines may be better stabilized with a 3.5-mm reconstruction plate or low contact-dynamic compression (LC-DC)-type plate (**Fig. 11**).

With Maisonneuve injuries, the author prefers plate fixation for fractures distal to the fibular neck because fibular length and rotation are restored. Alternatively, fibular length and rotation can be provisionally restored with a small pointed reduction forceps inserted through stab incisions in the lateral malleolus. Longitudinal traction and internal rotation forces are applied to the fibula as it is stabilized to the distal tibia and definitive syndesmotic fixation placed. Because of the gross instability associated with this pattern, medial and posterior fixation should be obtained where possible (**Fig. 12**).[20]

Decisionmaking with the Posterior Malleolus

There remains no consensus as to the minimum size of a posterior malleolar fragment necessitating fixation. As a general rule, however, fragments involving 25% or more of the tibial articular surface are associated with posterior instability and require stabilization. Restoration of fibular length should indirectly reduce the posterior malleolus,

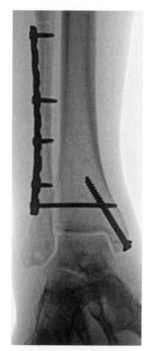

Fig. 11. Reconstruction plate and syndesmosis screw fixation for pronation-external rotation pattern.

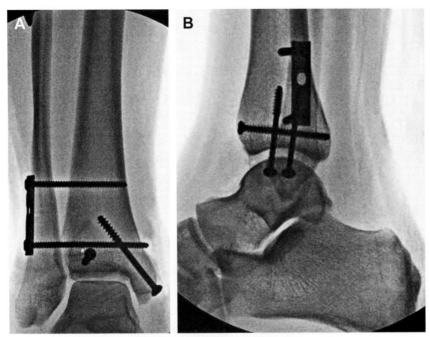

Fig. 12. Fixation for Maisonneuve injury: *A*) Medial and posterior fixation; *B*) Three-hole 1/3 tubular plate for washer effect laterally.

such that the fragment can be provisionally stabilized with 1.6-mm Kirschner wires (K-wires), and definitive cortical lag screw fixation placed percutaneously. The author prefers anterior to posterior screw fixation, starting anteromedially and aiming posterolaterally. Alternatively, posterior to anterior fixation can be used, although limb positioning typically makes this option more technically demanding.

Syndesmotic Instability

Considerable controversy continues to surround syndesmotic instability. In a cadaveric model, Boden and colleagues[21] described a critical transition zone between 3.0 and 4.5 cm proximal to the ankle mortise. With a tear of the deep deltoid ligament where medial fixation was not possible, syndesmosis fixation was necessary if the fibula fracture was proximal to this transition zone; conversely, if the deltoid ligament remained intact and medial fixation was possible, syndesmosis fixation was not necessary. Recent studies have suggested that these criteria are not entirely correct.

With the combination medial variant,[5] in which there is tension failure of the deep deltoid ligament and an avulsion fracture of the anterior colliculus, syndesmotic instability may remain despite fixation of anterior colliculus. Stark and colleagues[22] identified residual syndesmotic instability in 39% of supination-external rotation type IV patterns with a deltoid ligament injury following rigid lateral fixation (**Fig. 13**). These fractures were distal to the transition zone and therefore should not have required syndesmosis fixation. Thus, because of the variability in syndesmotic instability, all supination-external rotation, pronation-abduction, and pronation-external rotation patterns require an intraoperative external rotation stress test following definitive fracture fixation to assess for residual syndesmotic instability.

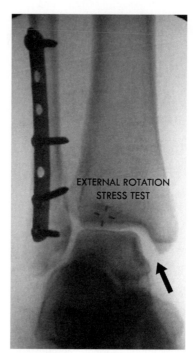

Fig. 13. Syndesmotic instability in S-ER IV pattern following fibular stabilization. Note widening of medial clear space with external rotation (*arrow*).

Syndesmotic Fixation

Similar controversy surrounds syndesmosis fixation (**Table 1**). There is currently no consensus about the optimum method of stabilization, position of the ankle during implant placement, weight-bearing restrictions, or need for and timing of implant removal. Screw fixation currently remains the gold standard and should be placed as position screws rather than as lag screws. Reduction of the syndesmosis must therefore be obtained before implant placement – a large pelvic clamp is invaluable in obtaining the reduction. A 1.6mm K-wire can be placed across and parallel to the plane of the syndesmosis before tightening of the pelvic clamp to prevent anterior or posterior translation of the fibula within the incisura fibularis (**Fig. 14**). McBryde and colleagues[23] defined the optimum location and trajectory for screw fixation of the syndesmosis as 2.0 cm proximal to the ankle mortise angling 30 degrees from posterolateral to anteromedial in the axial plane, and parallel to the ankle joint in the coronal plane. The surgeon should also have a low threshold for a medial arthrotomy in the event of an incomplete reduction, particularly in those patterns with a deltoid ligament injury as soft tissue interposition can prohibit reduction of the syndesmosis.

The author prefers obtaining medial and posterior fixation wherever possible, as this may obviate the need for syndesmotic fixation or at least increase the overall stability of the construct. I use a large pelvic clamp and k-wire to obtain a reduction; I use 3.5mm cortical screws placed through a 2-hole or 3-hole 1/3 tubular plate that functions as a washer to distribute stresses away from the screwhead, and I place the screws across all four cortices; and I perform an external-rotation stress test before and after implant placement (**Fig. 12**).

Table 1
Controversies in Syndesmotic Fixation

Controversies in Syndesmotic Fixation
3.5 mm versus 4.0 mm versus 4.5 mm cortical screws
3-cortices versus 4-cortices
One screw versus two screws
Screws through or outside of a plate
Bioresorbable screws
Suture anchors or tendon graft
Suture and washer device
Position of foot during implant placement
Length of weight-bearing restrictions
Need for and timing of implant removal

POSTEROMEDIAL VARIANT PATTERNS

Not every fracture is classifiable by the Lauge-Hansen classification. Atypical posteromedial variant patterns have been described; the incidence of these variant fractures ranges from 6%–11%, and have been associated with both high-energy and low-energy injury mechanisms.[24–27] These patterns feature a supination-external rotation or pronation-external rotation pattern with the fibula laterally, and a vertical split through the posterior colliculus with posteromedial subluxation of the talus, suggesting forced plantarflexion of an externally rotated talus within the ankle mortise. The vertical shear pattern posteromedially produces a double contour sign radiographically (**Fig. 15**)[24] and is an indication for a CT scan (**Fig. 16**). There is often variability with the fracture pattern posteriorly, ranging from a single fragment which includes the entire posterior malleolus, to separate posteromedial and posterolateral fragments.[25,27] Marginal impaction may also be present, particularly with higher energy injuries.[24]

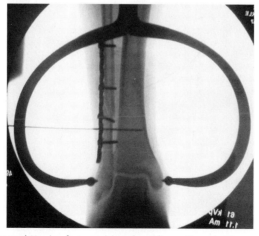

Fig. 14. Pelvic clamp and K-wire for provisional syndesmotic reduction.

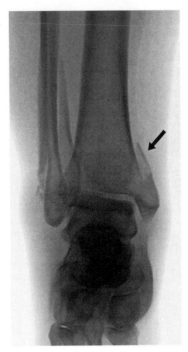

Fig. 15. Double contour sign (*arrow*) in atypical posteromedial variant pattern.

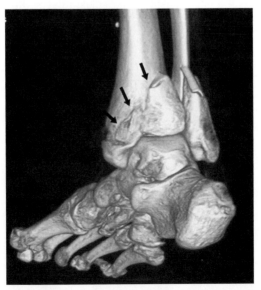

Fig. 16. 3-D CT scan of atypical posteromedial variant. Note large posteromedial fragment (*arrows*).

Fixation of unstable malleolar fractures typically begins with the fibula. With posteromedial variant patterns, however, the posteromedial subluxation of the talus can make intraoperative assessment of fibular length difficult, particularly in the instance of poor bone quality or fibular comminution. In this instance, failure of restoration of fibular length will also likely result in residual shortening of the posteromedial fragment and thus residual posteromedial subluxation of the talus (**Fig. 17**).

Weber[24] described a technique using a posterolateral approach in the prone position. The author prefers a posteromedial approach in the supine position through the floor of the posterior tibial tendon sheath.[27] The apex of the vertical spike is identified and buttress plate fixation is used, which should resolve the posteromedial subluxation of the talus and typically restores fibular length indirectly. The fibula is then stabilized, followed by medial fixation and supplemental lag screw fixation for the posterolateral portion of the posterior malleolus (**Fig. 18**).

POSTOPERATIVE PROTOCOLS

The author prefers splint immobilization for 2 weeks after surgery for all ankle fractures. The limb is then placed in an elastic compression stocking and prefabricated fracture boot and early range of motion exercises are begun. For simple patterns, the patient remains nonweight-bearing for 6 weeks postoperatively, and transitions to regular shoe-wear thereafter. Serial weight-bearing radiographs are obtained for at least 6 months postoperatively. I do not routinely remove hardware unless it is symptomatic, and in that instance not before 9–12 months following surgery.

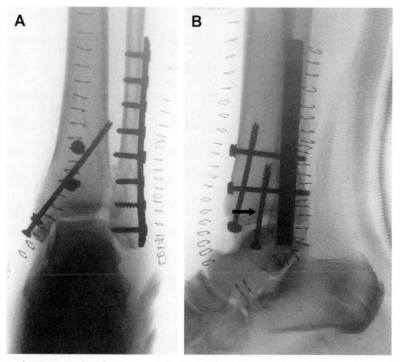

Fig. 17. *A)* Attempted reduction and fixation of atypical posteromedial variant pattern. *B)* Note residual shortening of posteromedial fragment and subluxation of talus (*arrow*).

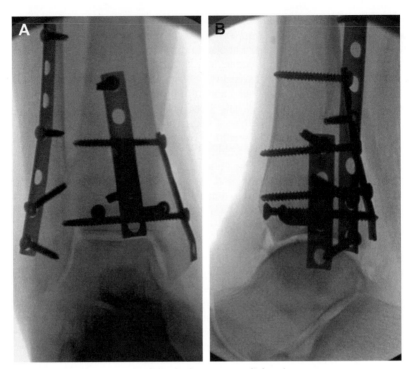

Fig. 18. *A, B*) Definitive fixation of atypical posteromedial variant pattern.

For fracture patterns requiring syndesmosis fixation, the patient is kept nonweight-bearing for 10 weeks postoperatively. In this instance, screw loosening and/or breakage is anticipated. Serial weight-bearing radiographs are obtained for at least 12 months postoperatively. I do not routinely remove syndesmosis screws unless symptomatic, and in that instance, not before 12 months following surgery.

For posteromedial variant patterns, the patient is similarly kept nonweight-bearing for 10 weeks postoperatively. Because of the extent of the posterior injury, aggressive ankle range of motion is emphasized, particularly ankle dorsiflexion. Serial weight-bearing radiographs are obtained for at least 12 months postoperatively. I do not routinely remove hardware unless it is symptomatic, and not before 12 months following surgery.

SUMMARY

Ankle fractures involve a spectrum of injury patterns from simple to complex, such that they are not always "just an ankle fracture." By combining the injury mechanism and the radiographic findings, the surgeon can apply the Lauge-Hansen classification in taking a rational approach to the management of these fractures. Syndesmotic instability and atypical patterns are becoming increasingly recognized, in part through the judicious use of CT scans. The goal of surgical stabilization includes atraumatic soft tissue management, rigid internal fixation, and early range of motion exercises in maximizing return of function.

REFERENCES

1. Phillips WA, Schwartz HS, Keller CS, et al. A prospective, randomized study of the management of severe ankle fractures. J Bone Joint Surg Am 1985;67: 67–78.
2. Ramsey PL, Hamilton W. Changes in tibiotalar area of contact caused by lateral talar shift. J Bone Joint Surg Am 1976;58:356–7.
3. Thordarson DB, Motamed S, Hedman T, et al. The effect of fibular malreduction on contact pressures in an ankle fracture malunion model. J Bone Joint Surg Am 1997;79:1809–15.
4. Lauge-Hansen N. Fractures of the ankle. II. combined experimental-surgical and experimental-produced fractures and roentgenologic investigation. Arch Surg 1950;60:957–85.
5. Tornetta P III. Competence of the deltoid ligament in bimalleolar ankle fractures after medial malleolus fixation. J Bone Joint Surg Am 2000;82:843–8.
6. McConnell T, Tornetta P III. Marginal plafond impaction in association with supination-adduction ankle fractures: a report of eight cases. J Orthop Trauma 2001;15: 447–9.
7. Egol KA, Amirtharage M, Tejwani NC, et al. Ankle stress test for predicting the need for surgical fixation of isolated fibular fractures. J Bone Joint Surg Am 2004;86:2393–8.
8. McConnell T, Creevy W, Tornetta P III. Stress examination of supination-external rotation-type fibular fractures. J Bone Joint Surg Am 2004;86:2171–8.
9. DeAngelis NA, Eskander MS, French BG. Does medial tenderness predict deep deltoid ligament incompetence? J Orthop Trauma 2007;21:244–7.
10. Michelson JD, Varner KE, Checcone M. Diagnosing deltoid injury in ankle fractures: the gravity stress view. Clin Orthop Relat Res 2001;387:178–82.
11. Gill JB, Risko T, Raducan V, et al. Comparison of manual and gravity stress radiographs for the evaluation of supination-external rotation fibular fractures. J Bone Joint Surg Am 2007;89:994–9.
12. Schock HJ, Pinzur M, Manion L, et al. The use of gravity or manual stress radiography in the assessment of supination-external rotation fractures of the ankle. J Bone Joint Surg Br 2007;89:1055–9.
13. Perren SM. Basic aspects of internal fixation. In: Müller ME, Allgöwer M, Schneider R, Willenegger H, editors. Manual of internal fixation. 3rd edition. New York: Springer-Verlag; 1991. p. 1–112.
14. Mast J. Preoperative planning and principles of reduction. In: Müller ME, Allgöwer M, Schneider R, Willenegger H, editors. Manual of internal fixation. 3rd edition. New York: Springer-Verlag; 1991. p. 159–76.
15. Schaffer JJ, Manoli AM. The antiglide plate for distal fibula fixation. A biomechanical comparison with fixation with a lateral plate. J Bone Joint Surg Am 1987;69: 596–604.
16. Winkler B, Weber BG, Simpson LA. The dorsal antiglide plate in the treatment of Danis-Weber type B fractures of the distal fibula. Clin Orthop Relat Res 1990;259: 204–9.
17. Lamontagne J, Blachut PA, Broekhuyse HM, et al. Surgical treatment of a displaced lateral malleolus fracture: the antiglide technique versus lateral plate fixation. J Orthop Trauma 2002;16:498–502.
18. Minihane KP, Lee C, Ahn C, et al. Comparison of lateral locking plate and antiglide plate for fixation of distal fibular fractures in osteoporotic bone: a biomechanical study. J Orthop Trauma 2006;20:562–6.

19. Weber M, Krause F. Peroneal tendon lesions caused by antiglide plates used for fixation of lateral malleolar fractures: the effect of plate and screw position. Foot Ankle Int 2005;26:281–5.

20. Gardner MJ, Brodsky A, Briggs SM, et al. Fixation of posterior malleolar fractures provides great syndesmotic stability. Clin Orthop Relat Res 2006;447:165–74.

21. Boden SD, Labropoulus PA, McGowin P, et al. Mechanical considerations for the syndesmosis screw: a cadaver study. J Bone Joint Surg Am 1989;71:1548–55.

22. Stark E, Tornetta P III, Creevy WR. Syndesmotic instability in Weber B ankle fractures: a clinical evaluation. J Orthop Trauma 2007;21:643–6.

23. McBryde A, Chiasson B, Wilhelm A, et al. Syndesmotic screw placement: a biomechanical analysis. Foot Ankle Int 1997;18:262–6.

24. Weber M. Trimalleolar fractures with impaction of the posteromedial tibial plafond: implications for talar stability. Foot Ankle Int 2004;25:716–27.

25. Haraguchi N, Haruyama H, Toga H, et al. Pathoanatomy of posterior malleolar fractures of the ankle. J Bone Joint Surg Am 2006;88:1085–92.

26. Gardner MJ, Boraiah S, Hentel KD, et al. The hyperplantarflexion ankle fracture variant. J Foot Ankle Surg 2007;46:256–60.

27. Clare MP. A typical osteoporotic malleolar fractures: Results of a specific treatment protocol. Presented at the American Orthopaedic Foot and Ankle Society 23rd Annual Summer Meeting. Toronto, Ontario, Canada, July 13–15, 2007.

Injuries to the Distal Tibiofibular Syndesmosis: an Evidence-Based Approach to Acute and Chronic Lesions

Stefan Rammelt, MD, PhD*, Hans Zwipp, MD, PhD, René Grass, MD, PhD

KEYWORDS

• Ankle • Syndesmosis • Biomechanics • Stability • Treatment

Syndesmotic injuries are estimated to occur in about 1% to 18% of all ankle sprains and are a common source of prolonged ankle pain and arthritis in athletes, especially if undiagnosed at first presentation.[1–7] The diagnosis of syndesmotic injury is not always easy because isolated sprains may be missed in the absence of a frank diastasis and syndesmotic instability may go unnoticed in the presence of bimalleolar ankle fractures. The prevalence of these injuries, therefore, may be higher than previously reported, as is also reflected in a high prevalence of late calcifications (up to 32%) at the syndesmosis in professional football players[8,9] and in an increasing amount of patients presenting with chronic instability.[6,10,11]

The syndesmotic complex provides a dynamic support to the ankle that is essential for normal performance. In 1773, the British surgeon Bromfeild[12] brought attention to the importance of a ligamentous junction between the distal tibia and fibula and speculated that if the distal fibula were part of the tibia, then after a few steps, a malleolar fracture would result. In the nineteenth century, the pathomechanical investigations of Maisonneuve[13] and Hönigschmied[14] shed light on the close connection between malleolar fractures and ligamentous injuries. Several investigators described bony avulsions of the anterior and posterior tibiofibular ligaments produced experimentally. At the beginning of the twentieth century, Chaput,[15] in 1907, described the "ligne claire" (tibiofibular clear space; TCS) as a measure for syndesmotic integrity, and Quénu,[16] in the same year, reported on a tibiofibular disatasis resulting from syndesmosis rupture.

Klinik und Poliklinik für Unfall und Wiederherstellungschirurgie, Universitätsklinikum, "Carl Gustav Carus" der TU Dresden, Fetscherstrasse 74, 01307 Dresden, Germany
* Corresponding author.
E-mail address: strammelt@hotmail.com (S. Rammelt).

Foot Ankle Clin N Am 13 (2008) 611–633
doi:10.1016/j.fcl.2008.08.001
1083-7515/08/$ – see front matter © 2008 Elsevier Inc. All rights reserved.

foot.theclinics.com

Both found malleolar fractures with diastasis to carry a worse prognosis than those without. Despite—or possibly because—of the centennial preoccupation of surgeons worldwide with syndesmotic injuries at the ankle, controversy prevails on several aspects of their management. Because there is some confusion regarding the anatomic terms and the biomechanical importance of the several parts of the syndesmotic complex, this article reviews the complex anatomy and pathomechanics before giving an evidence-based approach on the treatment of acute and chronic syndesmotic lesions.

ANATOMY: SORTING THE TERMS

The strong ligamentous junction between the tibia and fibula consists of three parts: (1) the proximal tibiofibular syndesmosis, formed by the ligamentum capitis fibulae anterius and posterius; (2) the aponeurotic interosseous membrane (IOM); and (3) the important distal tibiofibular syndesmotic complex, which consists of five separate portions (**Fig. 1**A).

1. The anterior inferior tibiofibular ligament (AITFL) descends from the anterior tubercle (Tubercúle de Tillaux-Chaput, Chaput's tubercle) of the tibia to the anterior aspect of the distal fibula (Le Fort's or Wagstaffe's tubercle). It has an average length of 16 mm and a breadth of 16 mm at the tibial origin and of 13 mm at the fibular insertion. Its average stiffness is about 5 kg/mm.[17] It consists of two to three portions running parallel to each other that are separated by gaps of less than 2 mm. The AITFL is tensioned maximally during plantarflexion.
2. The posterior inferior tibiofibular ligament (PITFL) is the strongest part of the distal syndesmosis. It descends posterolaterally from the posterior tubercle of the tibia. It is more compact and runs more horizontally than the AITFL.[18] Like the AITFL, it has a stiffness of 5 kg/mm, but the load to failure (120 kg in men, 70 kg in women) supersedes that of the AITFL (95 kg in men, 60 kg in women) in biomechanical testing.[17] Its average length is 20 mm, with an average width of 18 mm at the tibial origin and of 12 mm at the fibular insertion. The PITFL is under maximum tension during ankle dorsiflexion.[19]
3. The transverse tibiofibular ligament (TTFL) lies distal to the posterior tibiofibular ligament and has a fibrocartilagineous appearance. It runs almost horizontally to the posterior tubercle of the fibula and is sometimes hard to discriminate from the posterior tibiofibular ligament. It has therefore synonymously been described as a deep portion of the PITFL or a fibrocartilaginous reinforcement of the posterior capsule of the ankle joint.[18,20]
4. The interosseous tibiofibular ligament (IOL) is a mechanically important ligament that also contains elastic fibers and serves as buffer and stabilizer of the distal tibiofibular joint.[21,22] It has short and strong fibers that fan out into a network, almost completely filling the space between the distal tibia and fibula.[18] In the sagittal plane, it forms a triangle with its base 1 to 1.5 cm above the ankle joint level (see **Fig. 1**B). It lies in the pivot of the rotational plane of the distal fibula.[23,24] Synonyms include syndesmotic plate and ligamentum malleoli lateralis intermedium.[21,23]
5. The distal portion of the IOM consists of aponeurotic fibers that are recruited from the cranial origins of the anterior and posterior tibiofibular ligaments. It is in direct continuation of the apex of the pyramid-shaped IOL beginning 4 to 5 cm above the ankle joint level. Its fibers are thinner and longer than those of the IOL.

A direct contact area between the distal tibia and fibula was described by the anatomists of the nineteenth century.[20] In a recent anatomic study, Bartoniček[18] identified such a direct contact area in 23 of 30 cadaver ankles. This direct contact area has the

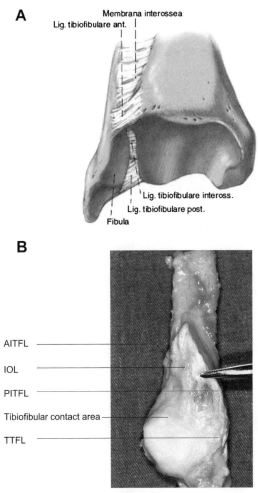

Fig. 1. Anatomy of the distal tibiofibular syndesmosis. (*A*) Seen from below are the ligamentum tibiofibulare anterius (anterior inferior tibiofibular ligament), posterius (posterior inferior tibiofibular ligament), and interosseum (interosseous tibiofibular ligament) and the membrana interossea cruris (IOM). (*From* Grass R, Zwipp H. Peroneus longus tenodesis for chronic instability of the distal tibiofibular syndesmosis. Operat Orthop Traumatol 2003;15(2):211; with permission.) (*B*) An anatomic specimen of the distal fibula seen from medial shows the triangular insertion of the IOL and the insertion points of the other syndesmotic ligaments and the semilunate contact zone between the distal tibia and fibula.

appearance of a small sickle-shaped joint facet covered with cartilage on both sides in the central part of the lower end of the fibular incision, directly below the IOL (see **Fig. 1**B). The anterior part of that contact area is filled with a triangular strip of fatty tissue, whereas the posterior part contains a richly vascularized V-shaped fibrous plica that is constantly observed.[23]

The incisura fibularis (peroneal groove) of the tibia has a varying appearance. In a cadaveric study, only 75% of the specimens had a concave surface of the lateral aspect of the tibia, 16% had a convex surface, and the remainder could not be classified due to an irregular shape.[24] Exact reduction of the fibula into the incisura may be hampered in the latter two groups. A more recent study[25] confirmed these results and found the fibular incisura to be significantly concave in 60% (more than 4 mm over the depth of the fibular incision) and shallowly concave in 40% of 20 cadaver limbs. The absolute depth of the incision varies considerably between 1.0 and 7.5 mm.[24]

RELEVANT ASPECTS OF ANKLE BIOMECHANICS

With normal stance, almost no twisting and shearing forces act on the ankle joint, and the pressures distributed through the joint surfaces are equal to the body weight.[19] Therefore, minimal tension is exerted on the tibiofibular ligaments under static conditions.[17,19] With axial loading of the ankle in neutral position, the PITFL is tensioned more than the AITFL, whereas both ligaments are tensioned by a 10° dorsiflexion even without axial load.[19] During normal gait, 10% to 17% of the body weight is taken up by the distal fibula,[26,27] which is substantially reduced after dissection of the syndesmosis and IOM.[28,29]

Because of its slightly oblique axis and the irregular shape of the talus, which is not cylindric but broader ventrally and laterally, the ankle joint is not a hinge joint.[30,31] A considerable clearance takes place between the talus and the distal fibula, which is limited by the tibiofibular syndesmosis.[29] The deep portion of the deltoid ligament also contributes to syndesmotic stability, acting as a restraint against lateral shift of the talus.[32,33]

The pivot of the ankle joint runs from the tip of the lateral malleolus to the tip of the medial malleolus and ascends 8° in the frontal plane and 6° in the transverse plain. The lateral slope of the talar dome is perpendicular to the pivot, whereas the medial side is inclined by 6°, which leads to a "pseudorotation" of the talus during movement in the ankle mortise.[30,31] Because of the dynamic fixation of the distal fibula to the distal tibia provided by the tibiofibular syndesmosis, the distal fibula performs a three-dimensional movement during physiologic dorsiflexion and plantarflexion at the ankle joint.[1,29,31,34,35]

With an intact syndesmosis, the intermalleolar distance increases with dorsiflexion of the talus by 1.0 to 1.25 mm, whereas the fibula rotates by 2° degrees externally.[1,29] During normal gait, the distal fibula translates about 2.4 mm distally and moves less than 0.2 to 0.4 mm anteroposteriorly.[31,34] A radiostereometric analysis of normal ankles demonstrated that under a physiologic external rotation momentum of 7.5 Newtonmeter (Nm) the fibula rotates externally between 2° and 5° and translates medially between 0 and 2.5 mm and posteriorly between 1 and 3.1 mm.[35]

SECTIONING STUDIES: WHAT PRODUCES SYNDESMOTIC INSTABILITY?

Several authors have demonstrated that complete sectioning of the AITFL results in pathologic external rotation of the talus. Sarsam and Hughes[32] found a 30° and 40° increase in external rotation of the talus through sectioning the AITFL after an experimental fibular fracture above and below the syndesmosis, respectively. Ogilvie-Harris and collaborators[36] found that the AITFL provided 35%, the TTFL 33%, the IOL 22%, and the PITFL 9% of the overall tibiofibular stability in a sectioning study. They concluded that with the rupture of two of these ligaments, relevant mechanical laxity would result. Xenos and colleagues[33] performed serial sectioning of the syndesmosis from anterior to posterior. Dissection of the AITFL alone resulted in an average 2.3-mm increase of the tibiofibular diastasis under a constant external rotation load of 5 Nm on the foot. Sectioning of the distal 8 cm of the IOM resulted in an additional increase of

2.2 mm, and sectioning of the PITFL resulted in another 2.8 mm increase, adding to an overall diastasis of 7.3 mm after sectioning of all syndesmotic ligaments. In addition, an average increase of 10.2° in external rotation of the talus was observed after sectioning of all ligaments. In this study, however, no specific reference was given to the IOL and the TTFL. These ligaments were presumably sectioned together with the distal IOM and the PITFL, respectively. Two studies[17,37] found greater strength of the PITFL compared with the AITFL (although not significantly greater) in 10 specimens.

Few studies have explicitly investigated the role of the IOL, although this ligament has long been believed by several investigators[1,22,38] to be the primary bond between the distal tibia and fibula. Only recently have experimental data highlighted the importance of an intact IOL for overall stability of the syndesmosis complex. Preliminary results from the authors' group[39] in 37 fresh frozen cadaver ankles demonstrated significant mortise widening by introducing a modified laminar spreader with a defined force of 15 kg only after dissection of the IOL after all other components of the syndesmosis complex had been dissected (**Fig. 2**). Hoefnagels and colleagues[40] demonstrated the significantly superior stiffness and load to failure of the IOL over the AITFL in 12 paired fresh frozen cadaver feet.

Biomechanical studies have shown that a lateral translation of 1 to 2 mm, shortening of 2 mm, and an external rotation of 5° of the distal fibula result in nonphysiologic pressure redistribution at the ankle joint.[41–43] A syndesmotic insufficiency with tibiofibular diastasis of more than 2 mm compared with the uninjured side may therefore be considered a prearthritic deformity (**Fig. 3**). This idea could be supported by the observation that among 64 consecutive patients who presented at the authors' clinic for ankle arthrodesis because of otherwise intractable arthritis after fracture-dislocations of the ankle, 13 (20.3%) had significant widening of the ankle mortise.[44]

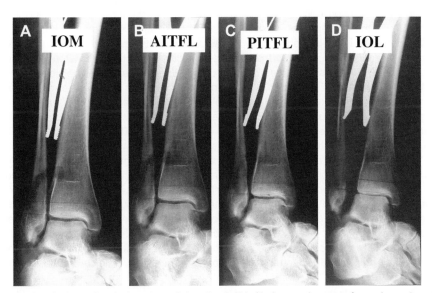

Fig. 2. (*A–D*) Biomechanical testing of the distal tibiofibular syndesmosis from the series of Bachmann and colleagues.[39] Frank diastasis occurred only after dissection of the IOL. It must be noted that the within the normal sequence with external rotation, the IOL ruptures before the PITFL. In pronation-abduction fractures, however, the intact IOL could preserve syndesmosis stability after rupture or avulsion of the AITFL and PITFL.[49]

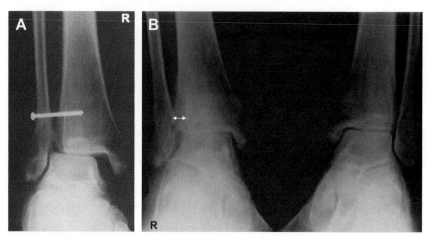

Fig. 3. (*A*) Obvious malreduction of a frank syndesmosis diastasis, with the screw impeding correct position of the fibula. (*B*) One year after screw removal, the patient presents with painful arthritis of the ankle with residual diastasis (*double arrow*), requiring arthrodesis.

MECHANISM OF INJURY

Syndesmotic injuries frequently occur in athletes, mostly in collision sports such as American football, hockey, rugby, wrestling, and lacrosse.[4,45–47] In these sports, the proportion of syndesmotic injuries among all ankle injuries is reported to rise up to 75% compared with 1% to 17% in the normal population.[3,45,46] Fritschy[48] noted a shift from lateral ankle sprains to syndesmotic injuries in skiing with the introduction of more firm skiing boots extending above the ankle. He observed 10 cases of syndesmotic injuries during a World Cup Slalom event when the inner ski was caught on a stake and the foot and ankle experienced forced external rotation within the boot.

Syndesmotic injury is produced by forced external rotation of the talus in the ankle mortise. Maisonneuve,[13] in 1840, produced distal fibular fractures ("fracture par divulsion") and syndesmosis ruptures with proximal fibular fractures by applying external rotation to the ankle. The latter were termed "fracture par diastase" and still bear his name. In 1877, Hönigschmied[14] was able to produce a variety of injuries by applying external rotation forces to 22 cadaver ankles, including complete diastasis of the syndesmosis in 8 cases or with rupture or avulsion of the AITFL, the IOL, or the PITFL (in 1 case) and the deltoid ligament (in 7 cases). Two injuries were purely ligamentous; in 2 cases, a fibular fracture was produced at 45 mm, 70 mm above the ankle joint. Two fractures of the proximal third of the fibula were seen, similar to those produced by Maisonneuve. An oblique fracture of the fibula (most likely a supination–external rotation injury) occurred in 12 cases. With the foot in dorsiflexion and pronation at the time of accident, the broader anterior part of the talus is forced into the ankle mortise, increasing the stress on the syndesmotic ligaments.[22,30,33,48–50] Even though this mechanism is well accepted in the literature and regularly found on taking the history of the accident, several other trauma mechanisms such as inversion and plantarflexion have been described.[4]

The sequelae of syndesmotic injury and associated fractures have been described extensively in the clinical and biomechanical series of Lauge-Hansen[49,51] in the midtwentieth century. With the foot in supination, external rotation leads to a rupture of the AITFL or leads to a bony avulsion at the anterior (Chaput's) tubercule on the anterior rim of the tibia or a Wagstaffe's/Le Fort's fragment at the fibular insertion of the AITFL.

With continuing external rotation, a spiral (Weber type B) fracture of the lateral malleolus follows. Even if external rotation is continued, the intact IOL, PITFL, and TTFL keep the correct tibiofibular relation proximal to the ankle joint.[49,52] The isolated rupture of the AITFL corresponds to a supination–external rotation stage I injury to the ankle, according to the Lauge-Hansen classification of ankle fractures.[49] Lauge-Hansen[53] termed isolated syndesmotic injuries "ligamentous ankle fractures."

With the foot in pronation, the deltoid ligament is tensioned and ruptures first; alternatively, a horizontal medial malleolar fracture occurs.[49] As external rotation continues, the AITFL and IOL rupture, followed by a spiral or oblique Weber type C fibular fracture; alternatively, a rupture of the IOM with a proximal fibular (Maisonneuve) fracture occurs. In stage IV, the PITFL and TTFL are ruptured or avulsed from the posterolateral rim of the tibia. With application of pure abduction force to the pronated foot, the medial malleolar fracture is followed by a rupture or avulsion of the AITFL and PITFL, whereas the IOL and IOM are stretched (stage II). If the force is continued, the distal fibula fractures indirectly at the level of the syndesmosis.[49]

Isolated complete ruptures and diastasis of the syndesmosis without a malleolar fracture are rare.[54] Most unstable syndesmotic lesions occur in the wake of pronation–external rotation stage III and IV injuries according to the Lauge-Hansen classification, which account for 8% to 11% of malleolar fractures and are associated with the highest rate of posttraumatic arthritis.[21,22,51] To a lesser degree, complete syndesmotic ruptures have to be suspected with pronation-abduction injuries.[49]

DIAGNOSIS

Patients who have acute or chronic syndesmotic injury present with pain in the anterolateral aspect of the ankle joint that is aggravated by forced dorsiflexion. The anterolateral aspect of the ankle is tender to palpation. With passive external rotation of the foot in neutral position against the fixed lower leg ("Frick's test," **Fig. 4**), pain over the syndesmosis can be provoked,[50] which has proved to be a sensitive test for syndesmotic injury in further studies.[8,44,55] Compressing the tibia to the fibula above the midpoint of the calf ("squeeze test") provokes pain at the level of the distal tibiofibular syndesmosis. This test has been described by Saunders[56] for fibular fractures and was later applied to syndesmotic injuries by Frick[50] and by Hopkinson and colleagues.[4] A variation of this test, the "cross-legged test," is performed by the patient.[57] The sitting patient rests the midtibia of the injured leg on the opposite

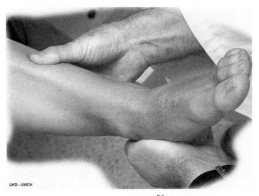

UKD - UWCH

Fig. 4. The external rotation test according to Frick[50] elicits pain at the level of the syndesmosis through external rotation of the foot with the lower leg fixed.

knee and produces a gentle downward force on the medial side of the knee. Pain in the region of the syndesmosis strongly suggests a syndesmotic injury. A functional "stabilization test" has been used by Amendola and collaborators,[47,58] mainly in athletes. A stabilizing athletic tape is applied tightly above the ankle joint and the patient is asked to stand, walk, and perform a toe raise and jump. If these maneuvers produce less pain after taping relative to before taping, the test is considered positive and the diagnosis of a syndesmosis sprain is confirmed.

So far, only the external rotation test has been shown to correlate with a syndesmotic injury and longer return to preinjury activities.[55,59] Biomechanical evaluation of the four common clinical tests showed that accurate prediction of the degree of mechanical injury is not possible with clinical testing alone.[60]

Standard radiographs of the ankle, including the "true" anteroposterior (AP) view and the mortise view, rule out malleolar fractures. A useful tool in detecting syndesmotic diastasis is the evaluation of the "espace clair" (TCS) according to Chaput,[15] which is measured on both sides in the true AP or mortise view (**Fig. 5**). Other radiographic landmarks include the tibiofibular overlap (TFO) and the medial clear space. An AP view of the complete lower leg is done in the event of local tenderness to exclude a proximal fibular (Maisonneuve) fracture (see the clinical example in **Fig. 6**). Generally, a TCS of less than 6 mm or a TFO of 6 mm or more (or 42% of fibular width) in the AP view or greater than 1 mm in the mortise view is considered to be normal.[61] A cadaveric study by Ostrum and colleagues[62] revealed some sex-specific differences. According to their data, a TCS less than 5.2 mm in female patients or 6.47 mm in male patients and a TFO greater than 2.1 mm in female patients or 5.7 mm in male patients (24% of the fibular width) should be considered to be normal. In any case, the values should be compared with those on the uninjured side. Latent diastasis is proved with stress radiographs, under regional anesthesia if necessary (**Fig. 7**). External rotation stress is applied manually under fluoroscopy or by lateral shift with a standardized Telos device (Telos GmbH, Marburg, Germany) on radiographs. These examinations are also useful for evaluating chronic syndesmotic insufficiency.[63]

CT scanning is a more accurate method of detecting syndesmotic injuries, especially with diastases of 3 mm or less that may go undetected with plain AP and mortise view radiographs.[64–66] CT scanning of both ankles allows determination of fibular shift, rotation, and shortening and the exact location of bony avulsions. Care is taken to evaluate the fibular rotation and tibiofibular distance in the horizontal plane at exactly the same level as on the uninjured side (see the clinical examples in **Figs. 6** and **8**).

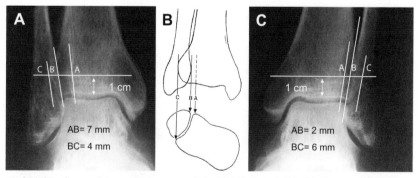

Fig. 5. (A–C) Radiographic measurements of the TCS (BC) and tibiofibular overlap (AB) in the AP view. With syndesmotic instability (*left image*), the clear space widens (diastasis) while the overlap is reduced.

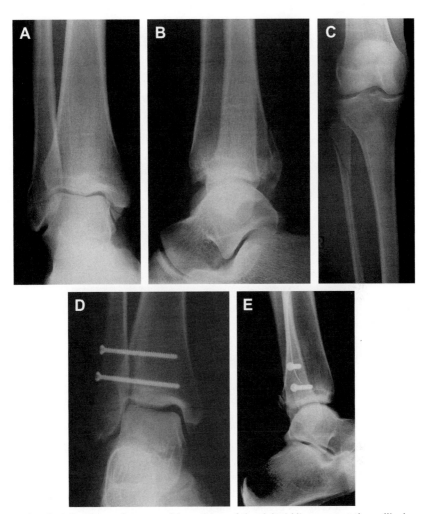

Fig. 6. (*A–C*) Maisonneuve fracture with avulsion of the deltoid ligament at the colliculus anterior, avulsion of the PITFL, tibiofibular diastasis, and high fibular fracture. (*D, E*) Open reduction and internal fixation is achieved with two syndesmosis screws. (*F–H*) Proper length and rotation of the fibula is measured with the respective CT reconstructions.

Coronal reconstruction allows exact determination of a lateral shift of the talus and measuring of the fibular length.[44] Generally, side-to-side differences of more than 2 mm are considered pathologic.[33,64]

MRI has been shown to effectively display the components of the syndesmotic complex with high interobserver agreement.[67] MRI has 93% specificity and 100% sensitivity for injury of the AITFL, and 100% specificity and sensitivity for injury of the PITFL compared with arthroscopy in acute injuries.[68] Sensitivity and specificity of MRI in chronic syndesmosis injury are 90% and 95%, respectively.[69]

CLASSIFICATION: IS IT OF ANY RELEVANCE?

Based on radiographic findings, Edwards and DeLee[54] classified traumatic syndesmotic sprains into latent diastasis (seen on stress radiographs only) and frank

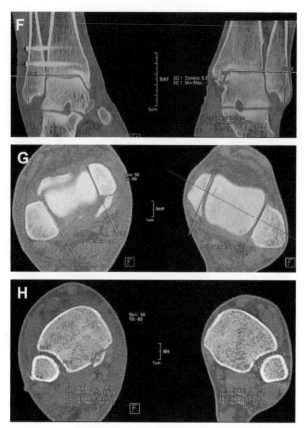

Fig. 6. (*continued*)

diastasis, which is obvious on plain radiographs. The latter was further divided by the investigators into four types based on the observation of just six cases, which fitted only two of these types. Because observations such as bowing of the fibula or wedging of the talus between the distal tibia and fibula are exceptionally rare without a fracture, the clinical relevance of such a classification system is highly questionable.

The West Point Ankle Grading System provided by Gerber and colleagues[3] distinguishes the following categories of pure ligamentous syndesmotic injuries: grade I—no evidence of instability (partial tear of the AITFL); grade II—no or slight evidence of instability (tear of the AITFL, partial tear of the IOL); and grade III—definite instability (complete tear of the syndesmotic ligaments). Again, the therapeutic consequences of introducing a grade II are not evident, and without arthroscopy or MRI, it may be impossible to discriminate between grades I and II. The investigators found no differences in outcome after functional treatment of grade I and II injuries.[3] Furthermore, the exact amount of injury and instability with "partial tears" remains unclear.

Because the existing classification systems do not offer a clear therapeutic algorithm, clinical and radiographic examination should focus on detecting and documenting the amount of latent and frank diastasis. The examiner should further discriminate between acute, subacute, and chronic sprains and atraumatic disorders of the soft tissues.

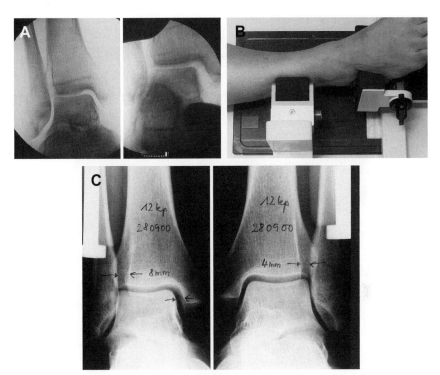

Fig. 7. Latent diastasis is detected with (*A*) external rotation under fluoroscopy or (*B*) standardized stress radiographs in a Telos device under regional anesthesia. (*C*) The latter is also useful to detect chronic syndesmotic insufficiency when comparing the measurements to the uninjured side. A side-to-side difference of more than 2 mm is considered pathologic.

In accordance with the existing biomechanical and clinical studies,[5,33,36,52,54] a frank or latent diastasis (as seen in stress films) of more than 2 mm compared with the uninjured side is highly suspicious of syndesmosis instability caused by a rupture of two or more ligaments and may lead to a pathologic alteration of ankle joint biomechanics. These injuries, which would be classified as grade III, should therefore be stabilized operatively.

TREATMENT AND RESULTS
Acute Syndesmosis Injury

Syndesmotic sprains without latent or frank diastasis ("high ankle sprains") are treated with a short course of rest, ice, elevation, and nonsteroidal anti-inflammatory medication (RICE) until subsidence of pain. This treatment may require 1 to 3 weeks' immobilization in a commercial brace or cast-boot.[47] In a second rehabilitation phase, physical therapy aims at restoring motion, strength, and function of the ankle.[3,45] Athletic activities are taken up again on an individual schedule. Advanced training is directed at returning to the preinjury sports level by increasing strength, neuromuscular control, and sport-specific tasks such as cutting, pivoting, and jumping.[47]

It should be noted that the average time lost from sports is longer and that residual complaints after 6 months are more frequent after syndesmotic sprains compared with lateral ankle sprains.[3,4,8,70] Overall, the results of nonoperative management of

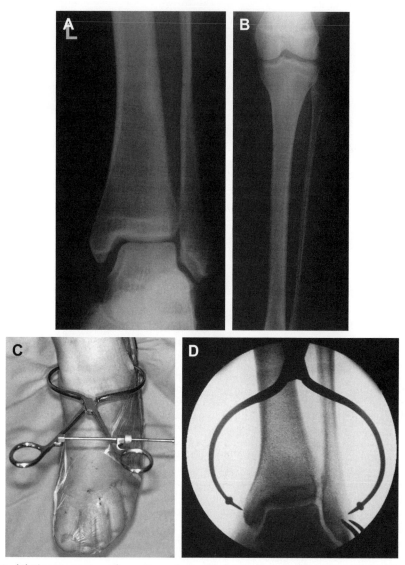

Fig. 8. (A) Ligamentous syndesmotic rupture with frank diastasis. (B) Because these injuries are rare, a high fibular fracture (Maisonneuve fracture) has to be ruled out. (C, D) The syndesmosis should be explored to allow proper reduction, which is achieved with a pelvic reduction clamp from the distal tibia to the distal fibula that lies exactly in the axis of the tibiotalar joint. Two syndesmosis screws are introduced within the axis of the reduction clamp. (E, F) Proper reduction of the fibula is ensured with axial and coronal CT, including the uninjured side.

syndesmosis sprains are favorable, with good to excellent outcomes in 86% to 100% and full return to sports in almost all cases.[3,7,70]

Cases of latent diastasis with isolated ruptures of the AITFL (grade II injuries) can be treated successfully with nonoperative treatment as described previously. The start of the second rehabilitation phase should be tailored to the patient's pain and functional

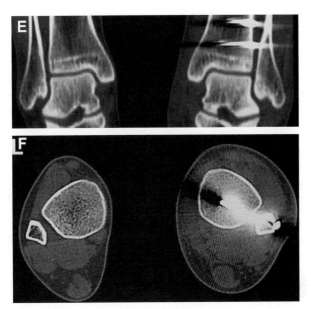

Fig. 8. (*continued*)

demand. Some investigators recommend more aggressive treatment in professional athletes, including arthroscopic debridement and percutaneous screw fixation;[47,58] however, this approach is not yet substantiated by biomechanical or clinical data.

Instability of the distal tibiofibular syndesmosis with a frank or latent diastasis of more than 2 mm, isolated or in conjunction with malleolar fractures, is treated with open reduction and fixation using one or two syndesmosis screws.[21,22,29,44,71] Boden and colleagues[72] defined the need to use a screw for syndesmotic stabilization from biomechanical studies. They concluded that a syndesmotic screw is warranted when the fibular fracture extends more than 4.5 cm above the ankle joint line. These criteria were validated in a clinical study done by the same group.[73] After open reduction and internal fixation of fibular fractures located more distally with questionable syndesmosis stability (mostly pronation-abduction fractures), stability of the syndesmotic complex is tested with a hook (Cotton test). It has to be borne in mind that syndesmotic instability leads to a posterior shift rather than a lateral shift of the fibula.[33] The fibula is therefore pulled laterally and dorsally, as described by Heim,[21] under fluoroscopic control. Alternatively, an intraoperative external rotation test is performed.[44] In cases of diastasis or AP instability of more than 2 mm, fixation with a syndesmosis screw is indicated.

In cases of pure ligamentous injury to the syndesmosis, percutanous reduction and stabilization has been described.[58] However, the authors' preference is to approach the distal tibiofibular syndesmosis directly from anterolateral to allow complete debridement of avulsed ligaments tissue or debris that may block proper reduction (see **Fig. 8**). The branches of the superficial peroneal nerve must be protected to avoid neuralgia. The fibular length is restored with a sharp reduction clamp pulling the tip of the fibula distally. Care is taken to position the fibula properly into the incisura fibularis of the tibia, which is best achieved with a bimalleolar (pelvic) reduction clamp (see **Fig. 8**). This clamp also provides the best position for the syndesmosis screw. The anterior rim of the fibula should align with Chaput's tubercule. When anatomic reduction of the syndesmosis is not possible by way of a lateral approach, the medial aspect of the ankle and the deltoid ligament should be explored with a small anteromedial approach. All ligamentous or capsular debris is removed. The necessity of a direct suture of a torn deltoid ligament, if detected, is not yet established. After proper reduction, the position of the fibula may be secured temporarily with a Kirschner wire.[44] The necessity of bringing the foot into dorsiflexion to ensure a correct tibiofibular distance[71,74] was challenged by cadaver experiments during which it appeared that overtightening of the syndesmosis was not a major concern.[75] The best position is probably with the ankle in neutral.

It is amazing how many biomechanical studies have been conducted to determine the exact number and size of the syndesmotic screws to assure solid tibiofibular fixation. From the existing data, there is no mechanical advantage of stainless steel over titanium screws,[76] 4.5-mm over 3.5-mm screws,[77,78] or quadricortical over tricortical screws.[76,79] Two 3.5-mm tricortical screws appear to provide more stability than a 4.5-mm quadricortical screw.[80] Bioabsorbable screws from polylactic acid have been used without side effects and with similar success rates to metallic screws in prospective clinical studies.[81–83] Seitz and colleagues[84] successfully used an endobutton suture technique that was shown to be biomechanically equivalent to a 4.5-mm quadricortical screw[85] and associated with faster rehabilitation in a clinical study.[86] Other semirigid fixation techniques have been reported anecdotally.[87] The use of two screws through a third-tubular plate was found to be useful in total ankle arthroplasty with syndesmosis fusion[88] but has not been shown to be mechanically superior in syndesmosis injuries.[89] There is general agreement that the screw should be positioned at an angle of approximately 30° from posterolateral to antermedial, thus being perpendicular to the fibular incisura within the distal tibia.[21,90] Placement of the screw within 2 cm of the tibiotalar joint line is associated with less widening than screw placement 3.5 cm above the joint line.[71]

In cases of syndesmosis rupture accompanied by a malleolar fracture, the authors' preference is to use a single 3.5-mm cortical screw positioned 2 cm above the joint level. The distal fibula is reduced into the tibial incisura with the help of a reduction clamp spanning from the midline of the distal fibula to that of the distal tibia at the joint level. The syndesmosis screw is then introduced exactly in the plane of the reduction clamp from posterolateral to anteromedial to ensure exact placement in the pivot of the distal fibula (which may differ from the frequently stated 30°) and penetrates three cortices. The screw is specifically not overdrilled so as to avoid any lag effect. The ruptured anterior tibiofibular ligament is sutured separately or reattached with a small or minifragment screw in cases of bony avulsion at the distal tibia or fibula. In cases of pure ligamentous syndesmosis rupture—including Maisonneuve injuries (see **Fig. 6**)—a second screw is introduced parallel to and above the first one to assure rotational stability.[44,91]

When reviewing CT scans with respect to syndesmotic reduction, Pottorff and Kaye[92] found the syndesmosis to be usually underreduced. Even with good-quality fluoroscopic or radiographic images, malreduction of the syndemosis may go undetected in as much as 24% of cases in clinical studies.[65,66] Compared with CT, the sensitivity and specificity of standard radiographs was found to be 31% and 83%, respectively,[66] which compares well to the preoperative measurements.[64] A postoperative CT scan of both ankles is therefore advocated after syndesmosis screw placement to ensure tibiofibular congruency and to allow early correction, if necessary.[65,93]

Syndesmosis screws are kept in place for 6 to 8 weeks.[21,22,44,47] During that time, the patient is restricted to 15 kg partial weight-bearing in a below-knee cast. Some investigators advocate removal of the screw (or screws) not before 3 months;[61,89,94] however, there is no clinical evidence of recurrence after 6 or 8 weeks of screw placement. If the screw is left in excessively long or permanently, then screw breakage and osteolysis around the screw is likely to occur while the ankle joint regains its physiologic tibiofibular clearance,[21,44,95] because the syndesmosis screw restricts normal ankle motion.[29]

Few small case series report the results after operative treatment of pure ligamantous syndesmotic injuries. Leeds and Ehrlich[52] and Fritschy[48] saw no recurrence after open reduction, screw fixation, and suture of the AITFL (and deltiod ligamant) in six and three cases, respectively.

In their classic study, Edwards and DeLee[54] looked at the 4-year results of 34 patients treated with bimalleolar and trimalleolar ankle fractures. They found significant correlations between the adequacy of syndesmosis reduction and arthritis at follow-up, between the accuracy of initial syndesmosis reduction and late stability, between late syndesmosis stability and the final outcome, and between the adequacy of the reduction of the lateral malleolus and that of the syndesmosis. These results suggest that adequacy of syndesmosis reduction is highly predictive of the late results in malleolar fractures. Chissell and Jones,[96] in a study of 43 patients who had Weber type C ankle fractures of which 31 were treated with a syndesmosis screw, showed that a syndesmotic widening of more than 1.5 mm was associated with an unacceptable outcome at 2 to 8 years' follow-up. Similarly, Kennedy and colleagues[97] reported a significant association between syndesmotic malreduction and poor outcomes. More recently, Weening and Bhandari[98] demonstrated that the only significant predictor of functional outcome as judged with validated scores after ankle fractures with transsyndesmotic screw fixation in 51 cases was reduction of the syndesmosis. Although several studies suggested an overuse of the syndesmosis screw,[73,96,98] this did not adversely affect the final result.

It follows clearly from the existing data that as long as the syndesmosis is reduced anatomically, either of the reported techniques leads to satisfactory results. Proper reduction of the fibula within the incisura fibularis is therefore the most important step while treating these injuries and should be confirmed with a postoperative CT scan or three-dimensional fluoroscopy, if available.

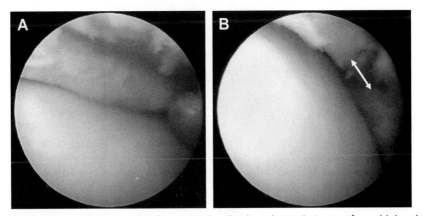

Fig. 9. (A) Hypertrophy and arthrofibrosis at the distal syndesmosis 1 year after a high ankle sprain without evidence of syndesmotic instability. (B) Arthroscopic treatment consists of arthrolysis and resection of the hypertrophied scar to improve ankle motion. The double arrow indicates the TCS.

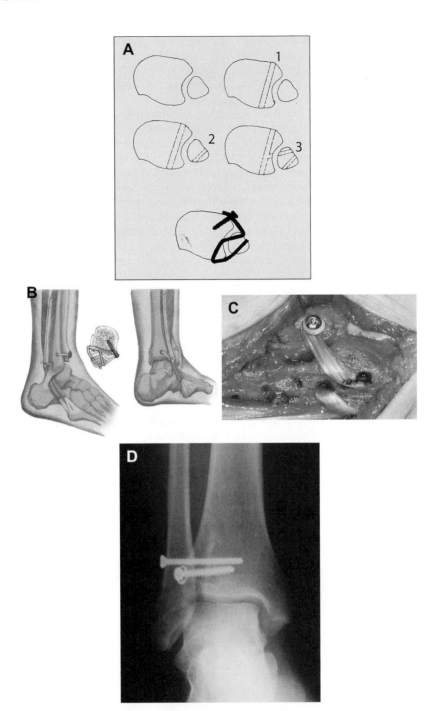

Several studies report the occurrence of heterotopic ossifications between the distal tibia and fibula after syndesmotic injury. Hopkinson and colleagues[4] found heterotopic ossifications in 9 of 10 cases on long-term evaluation; all were asymptomatic. On the other hand, McMaster and Scranton[99] found radiographic evidence of tibiofibular synostosis in seven patients who had persistent pain 3 to 11 months after a ligamentous syndesmosis injury. The first two patients had recurrent synostosis; the other five patients had no recurrence or pain at 28 months' follow-up after application of bone wax to the resection edges. Veltri and colleagues[100] reported 2 cases of symptomatic tibiofibular synostosis in collegiate and professional football players. After resection of the synostosis, both patients returned to full activity. Kaye[95] noted a tibiofibular synostosis in 4 of 30 cases following syndesmotic fixation. When a painful, complete synostosis occurs, it should be resected and the resection areas sealed with bone wax to avoid recurrence. In the authors' experience, asymptomatic synostoses frequently prove incomplete on CT scan and require no further treatment.

Chronic Syndesmotic Instability

As pointed out earlier, there is evidence from biomechanical and clinical studies that chronic syndesmotic instability with frank diastasis of more than 2 mm leads to altered joint mechanics, resulting in inferior clinical results and eventually posttraumatic arthritis.[5,33,43,54,95–97] Only a few articles, however, discuss options for surgical reconstruction for chronic instability after syndesmosis ruptures. Chronic syndesmotic instability is characterized by continued pain, limited range of motion, and the inability to perform on a preinjury level after syndesmosis injuries with or without malleolar fractures. Typically, patients report a sensation of giving way and pain while walking on uneven ground.[5,10] The clinical findings are less specific than with acute injury. Diagnosis is finally confirmed with weight-bearing and stress radiographs of both ankles.[5] Again, CT scans provide the best anatomic detail on the position of the fibula within the incisura, the presence of chronic bony avulsions, and deformities of the distal fibula after malleolar fracture.

Ogilvie-Harris and colleagues[6] performed arthroscopic treatment for chronic syndesmotic injuries in 19 patients after an average of 2 years of symptoms. Arthroscopic resection of the torn interosseous ligament and chondroplasty relieved symptoms in all patients in the short-term. This method, however, does not restore syndesmotic stability. It may be useful in achieving improved range of motion at the ankle after intra-articular adhesions following syndesmotic injury (**Fig. 9**). More recently, Han and colleagues[69] reported significant functional improvement from arthroscopic marginal resection of chronically injured syndesmosis ligaments irrespective of additional screw fixation, suggesting that hypertrophy and impingement are a main cause of pain in chronic syndesmotic injury.

Tibiofibular fusion with bone grafting, as recommended by several investigators,[38,89,101] produces a nonphysiologic stiffness of the ankle mortise, preventing the fibula from its normal movements described earlier, thus restricting talar

◀———————————————————————————————

Fig. 10. (*A, B*) Peroneus longus ligamentoplasty for chronic syndesmosis instability (same patient as in **Fig. 7**C). The split peroneus longus tendon is guided through the fibular and tibial channels to achieve a stable and dynamic three-strand support of the syndesmosis. (*From* Grass R, Zwipp H. Peroneus longus tenodesis for chronic instability of the distal tibiofibular syndesmosis. Operat Orthop Traumatol 2003;15(2):220; with permission). (*C*) A syndesmosis screw is introduced for 8 weeks until healing of the tendon. (*D*) The screw with washer in the anterior tubercle holds the graft and remains in place.

movement. Consequently, this procedure may lead to arthritis of the ankle.[102] Apart from a case report,[101] there are no reported results from clinical studies on tibiofibular fusion for chronic syndesmotic instability.

Mullins and Sallis[103] reported on the successful treatment of recurrent ankle sprains in the subacute and chronic stage with placement of a Johansen lag screw. Harper[11] performed delayed reduction and stabilization with a 6.5-mm cancellous screw, engaging four cortices for chronic syndesmotic instability. In a preliminary report, satisfactory results were obtained in five of six cases. Beumer and colleagues[10] treated 9 patients who had chronic syndesmotic instability (confirmed arthroscopically) with mobilization and refixation of the elongated AITFL with a 7 × 7-mm bone block. Syndesmosis fixation was achieved with a screw. At 45 months, all patients had improved without signs of instability. Wolf and Amendola[58] treated 14 patients who had chronic syndesmotic injury but not diastasis with arthroscopic debridement and percutaneous screw fixation for 8 to 10 weeks in case of latent instability. The short-term results were excellent in 2 patients, good in 10 patients, and fair in 4 patients.

Because the syndesmosis provides a dynamic support to the ankle joint, it would seem logical to search for a dynamic reconstruction of the chronically torn ligaments in cases of chronic syndesmotic insufficiency. Castaing and colleagues[104] performed reconstruction of the AITFL and PITFL with the peroneus brevis tendon guided through bony channels in the distal tibia and fibula. The authors modified this procedure to achieve a three-point fixation of the distal fibula[5] because of the previously mentioned experimental data that demonstrated the importance of the IOL for syndesmotic stability.[39,40] The ligamentoplasty uses half of the peroneus longus tendon, which is split from the distal tip of the fibula upward at a length of 18 cm. The split tendon is guided through one canal in the distal tibia parallel to the fibular incisura and two canals in the distal fibula lying at an angle of 45° to each other, thus paralleling the normal anatomic conditions of the syndesmotic complex (**Fig. 10**). The free end of the tendon is then secured with a 3.5-mm cancellous screw with a washer inserted obliquely to the tibial canal. A 3.5-mm syndesmosis screw is placed for 8 weeks as in acute syndesmotic ruptures. The first results in a series of 16 patients followed for an average of 18 months were encouraging, with 15 of 16 being relieved of pain and chronic instability.[5] The authors have meanwhile treated more than 80 patients with this method, and longer follow-up is pending. It appears from the existing data that patient compliance and the absence of symptomatic arthritis or bony defects at the time of diagnosis are preconditions for a good functional result. In cases of painful arthritis with chronic syndesmosis instability, ankle arthrodesis or tibiofibular fusion with total ankle arthroplasty should be considered.[88,105]

REFERENCES

1. Close JR. Some applications of the functional anatomy of the ankle joint. J Bone Joint Surg Am 1956;38:761–81.
2. Fallat L, Grimm DJ, Saracco JA. Sprained ankle syndrome: prevalence and analysis of 639 acute injuries. J Foot Ankle Surg 1998;37(4):280–5.
3. Gerber JP, Williams GN, Scoville CR, et al. Persistent disability associated with ankle sprains: a prospective examination of an athletic population. Foot Ankle Int 1998;19(10):653–60.
4. Hopkinson WJ, St Pierre P, Ryan JB, et al. Syndesmosis sprains of the ankle. Foot Ankle 1990;10(6):325–30.

5. Grass R, Rammelt S, Biewener A, et al. Peroneus longus ligamentoplasty for chronic instability of the distal tibiofibular syndesmosis. Foot Ankle Int 2003; 24(5):392–7.
6. Ogilvie-Harris DJ, Gilbart MK, Chorney K. Chronic pain following ankle sprains in athletes: the role of arthroscopic surgery. Arthroscopy 1997;13(5):564–74.
7. Amendola A, Williams G, Foster D. Evidence-based approach to treatment of acute traumatic syndesmosis (high ankle) sprains. Sports Med Arthrosc 2006; 14(4):232–6.
8. Boytim MJ, Fischer DA, Neumann L. Syndesmotic ankle sprains. Am J Sports Med 1991;19(3):294–8.
9. Vincelette P, Laurin CA, Lévesque HP. The footballer's ankle and foot. Can Med Assoc J 1972;107:872–7.
10. Beumer A, Heijboer RP, Fontijne WP, et al. Late reconstruction of the anterior distal tibiofibular syndesmosis: good outcome in 9 patients. Acta Orthop Scand 2000;71(5):519–21.
11. Harper MC. Delayed reduction and stabilization of the tibiofibular syndesmosis. Foot Ankle Int 2001;22(1):15–8.
12. Bromfeild W. Chirurgical observations and cases, vol. 2. London: Cadell; 1773.
13. Maisonneuve JGT. Recherches sur la fracture du peroné. Arch Gen de Med 1840;7(Sér 3):165–87 [In French].
14. Hönigschmied J. Leichenexperimente über die Zerreißung der Bänder am Sprunggelenk mit Rücksicht auf die Entstehung der indirekten Knöchelfrakturen. Dtsch Z Chir 1877;8:239–60 [In German].
15. Chaput V. Les fractures malléolaires du cou-de-pieds et les accidents du travail. Paris: Masson; 1907 [In French].
16. Quénu E. Du diastasis de l'articulation tibiopéronière inférieure. Rev Chir (Paris) 1907;35:897–944 [In French].
17. Sauer HD, Jungfer E, Jungbluth KH. Experimentelle Untersuchungen zur Reißfestigkeit des Bandapparates am menschlichen Sprunggelenk. Hefte Unfallheilkd 1978;131:37–42 [In German].
18. Bartoniček J. Anatomy of the tibiofibular syndesmosis and its clinical relevance. Surg Radiol Anat 2003;25(5–6):379–86.
19. Wruhs O, Habernek H, Franek F. Static stress of tibiofibular syndesmosis. Unfallchirurgie 1987;13(3):129–34 [in German].
20. Fick R. Handbuch der Anatomie und Mechanik der Gelenke unter Berücksichtigung der bewegenden Muskeln. Part I: Anatomie der Gelenke. Jena (LA): Fischer; 1904 [In German].
21. Heim U. Malleolar fractures. Unfallheilkunde 1983;86(6):248–58 [in German].
22. Zwipp H. Chirurgie des Fußes. Wien (NY): Springer-Verlag; 1994. [In German].
23. Lutz W. Zur Struktur der unteren Tibiofibularverbindung und der Membrana interossea cruris. Zeitschrift für Anatomie und Entwicklungsgeschichte 1942;111: 315–21 [In German].
24. Höcker K, Pachucki A. The fibular incisure of the tibia. The cross-sectional position of the fibula in distal syndesmosis. Unfallchirurgie 1989;92(8):401–6 [in German].
25. Ebraheim NA, Lu J, Yang H, et al. The fibular incisure of the tibia on CT scan: a cadaver study. Foot Ankle Int 1998;19(5):318–21.
26. Lambert KL. The weight-bearing function of the fibula. A strain gauge study. J Bone Joint Surg Am 1971;53(3):507–13.
27. Goh JC, Mech AM, Lee EH, et al. Biomechanical study on the load-bearing characteristics of the fibula and the effects of fibular resection. Clin Orthop Relat Res 1992;279:223–8.

28. Libotte M, Klein P, Colpaert H, et al. Biomechanical study of the ankle joint. Rev Chir Orthop Reparatrice Appar Mot 1982;68(5):299–305 [in French].

29. Peter RE, Harrington RM, Henley MB, et al. Biomechanical effects of internal fixation of the distal tibiofibular syndesmotic joint: comparison of two fixation techniques. J Orthop Trauma 1994;8(3):215–9.

30. Inman VT. The joints of the ankle. Baltimore (MD): Williams & Wilkins; 1976.

31. Reimann R, Anderhuber F. Kompensationsbewegungen der Fibula, die durch die Keilform der Torchlea tali erzwungen werden. Acta Anat 1980;108:60–7 [In German].

32. Sarsam IM, Hughes SP. The role of the anterior tibio-fibular ligament in talar rotation: an anatomical study. Injury 1988;19(2):62–4.

33. Xenos JS, Hopkinson WJ, Mulligan ME, et al. The tibiofibular syndesmosis. Evaluation of the ligamentous structures, methods of fixation, and radiographic assessment. J Bone Joint Surg Am 1995;77(6):847–56.

34. Scranton PE Jr, McMaster JG, Kelly E. Dynamic fibular function: a new concept. Clin Orthop Relat Res 1976;118:76–81.

35. Beumer A, Valstar ER, Garling EH, et al. Kinematics of the distal tibiofibular syndesmosis: radiostereometry in 11 normal ankles. Acta Orthop Scand 2003;74(3): 337–43.

36. Ogilvie-Harris DJ, Reed SC, Hedman TP. Disruption of the ankle syndesmosis: biomechanical study of the ligamentous restraints. Arthroscopy 1994;10(5):558–60.

37. Beumer A, van Hemert WL, Swierstra BA, et al. A biomechanical evaluation of the tibiofibular and tibiotalar ligaments of the ankle. Foot Ankle Int 2003;24(5): 426–9.

38. Outland T. Sprains and separations of the inferior tibiofibular joint without important fracture. Am J Surg 1943;59:320.

39. Bachmann L, Seifert C, Zwipp H. Experimental and clinical diagnosis of ankle injuries with the syndesmosis spreader. In: Schmidt R, Benesch S, Lipke K, editors. Chronic ankle instability. Ulm (Germany): Libri; 2000. p. 235–8.

40. Hoefnagels EM, Waites MD, Wing ID, et al. Biomechanical comparison of the interosseous tibiofibular ligament and the anterior tibiofibular ligament. Foot Ankle Int 2007;28(5):602–4.

41. Ramsey PL, Hamilton W. Changes in tibiotalar area of contact caused by lateral talar shift. J Bone Joint Surg Am 1976;58:356–7.

42. Zindrick MR, Hopkins DE, Knight GW, et al. The effect of lateral talar shift upon the biomechanics of the ankle joint. Orthopaedic Transactions 1985;9:332–3.

43. Thordarson DB, Motamed S, Hedman T, et al. The effect of fibular malreduction on contact pressures in an ankle fracture malunion model. J Bone Joint Surg Am 1997;79(12):1809–15.

44. Grass R, Herzmann K, Biewener A, et al. Injuries of the distal tibiofibular syndesmosis. Unfallchirurg 2000;103:520–32 [in German].

45. Nussbaum ED, Hosea TM, Sieler SD, et al. Prospective evaluation of syndesmotic ankle sprains without diastasis. Am J Sports Med 2001;29(1):31–5.

46. Wright RW, Barile RJ, Surprenant DA, et al. Ankle syndesmosis sprains in national hockey league players. Am J Sports Med 2004;32(8):1941–5.

47. Williams GN, Jones MH, Amendola A. Syndesmotic ankle sprains in athletes. Am J Sports Med 2007;35(7):1197–207.

48. Fritschy D. An unusual ankle injury in top skiers. Am J Sports Med 1989;17(2): 282–5 [discussion: 285–6].

49. Lauge-Hansen N. Fractures of the ankle II: combined experimental/surgical and experimental roentgenologic investigation. Arch Surg 1950;60:957–85.

50. Frick H. Diagnosis, therapy and results of acute instability of the syndesmosis of the upper ankle joint (isolated anterior rupture of the syndesmosis). Orthopäde 1986;15(6):423–6 [in German].
51. Lauge-Hansen N. Fractures of the ankle. IV. Clinical use of genetic roentgen diagnosis and genetic reduction. AMA Arch Surg 1952;64(4):488–500.
52. Leeds HC, Ehrlich MG. Instability of the distal tibiofibular syndesmosis after bimalleolar and trimalleolar ankle fractures. J Bone Joint Surg Am 1984;66(4):490–503.
53. Lauge-Hansen N. "Ligamentous" ankle fractures. Diagnosis and treatment. Acta Chir Scand 1949;97:544–50.
54. Edwards GS Jr, DeLee JC. Ankle diastasis without fracture. Foot Ankle 1984; 4(6):305–12.
55. Beumer A, Swierstra BA, Mulder PG. Clinical diagnosis of syndesmotic ankle instability: evaluation of stress tests behind the curtains. Acta Orthop Scand 2002;73(6):667–9.
56. Saunders EA. Ligamentous injuries of the ankle. Am Fam Physician 1980;22(2): 132–8.
57. Kiter E, Bozkurt M. The crossed-leg test for examination of ankle syndesmosis injuries. Foot Ankle Int 2005;26(2):187–8.
58. Wolf BR, Amendola A. Syndesmosis injuries in the athlete: when and how to operate. Curr Opin Orthop 2002;31:151–4.
59. Alonso A, Khoury L, Adams R. Clinical tests for ankle syndesmosis injury: reliability and prediction of return to function. J Orthop Sports Phys Ther 1998; 27(4):276–84.
60. Beumer A, van Hemert WL, Swierstra BA, et al. A biomechanical evaluation of clinical stress tests for syndesmotic ankle instability. Foot Ankle Int 2003;24(4): 358–63.
61. Harper MC, Keller TS. A radiographic evaluation of the tibiofibular syndesmosis. Foot Ankle 1989;10(3):156–60.
62. Ostrum RF, de Meo P, Subramanian R. A critical analysis of the anterior-posterior radiographic anatomy of the ankle syndesmosis. Foot Ankle Int 1995;16(3): 128–31.
63. Grass R, Zwipp H. Peroneus longus tenodesis for chronic instability of the distal tibiofibular syndesmosis. Oper Orthop Traumatol 2003;15(2):208–25.
64. Ebraheim NA, Lu J, Yang H, et al. Radiographic and CT evaluation of tibiofibular syndesmotic diastasis: a cadaver study. Foot Ankle Int 1997;18(11):693–8.
65. Barthel S, Grass R, Zwipp H. Stellenwert der Computertomographie bei der Evaluierung operativ versorgter Sprunggelenksfrakturen. Hefte Unfalchir 2002; 284:235–6 [In German].
66. Gardner MJ, Demetrakopoulos D, Briggs SM, et al. Malreduction of the tibiofibular syndesmosis in ankle fractures. Foot Ankle Int 2006;27(10):788–92.
67. Muhle C, Frank LR, Rand T, et al. Tibiofibular syndesmosis: high-resolution MRI using a local gradient coil. J Comput Assist Tomogr 1998;22(6):938–44.
68. Takao M, Ochi M, Oae K, et al. Diagnosis of a tear of the tibiofibular syndesmosis. The role of arthroscopy of the ankle. J Bone Joint Surg Br 2003;85(3):324–9.
69. Han SH, Lee JW, Kim S, et al. Chronic tibiofibular syndesmosis injury: the diagnostic efficiency of magnetic resonance imaging and comparative analysis of operative treatment. Foot Ankle Int 2007;28(3):336–42.
70. Taylor DC, Englehardt DL, Bassett FH 3rd. Syndesmosis sprains of the ankle. The influence of heterotopic ossification. Am J Sports Med 1992;20(2):146–50.
71. McBryde A, Chiasson B, Wilhelm A, et al. Syndesmotic screw placement: a biomechanical analysis. Foot Ankle Int 1997;18(5):262–6.

72. Boden SD, Labropoulos PA, McCowin P, et al. Mechanical considerations for the syndesmosis screw. A cadaver study. J Bone Joint Surg Am 1989;71(10): 1548–55.

73. Yamaguchi K, Martin CH, Boden SD, et al. Operative treatment of syndesmotic disruptions without use of a syndesmotic screw: a prospective clinical study. Foot Ankle Int 1994;15(8):407–14.

74. Olerud C. The effect of the syndesmotic screw on the extension capacity of the ankle joint. Arch Orthop Trauma Surg 1985;104(5):299–302.

75. Tornetta P 3rd, Spoo JE, Reynolds FA, et al. Overtightening of the ankle syndesmosis: is it really possible? J Bone Joint Surg Am 2001;83-A(4):489–92.

76. Beumer A, Campo MM, Niesing R, et al. Screw fixation of the syndesmosis: a cadaver model comparing stainless steel and titanium screws and three and four cortical fixation. Injury 2005;36(1):60–4.

77. Thompson MC, Gesink DS. Biomechanical comparison of syndesmosis fixation with 3.5- and 4.5-millimeter stainless steel screws. Foot Ankle Int 2000;21(9): 736–41.

78. Hansen M, Le L, Wertheimer S, et al. Syndesmosis fixation: analysis of shear stress via axial load on 3.5-mm and 4.5-mm quadricortical syndesmotic screws. J Foot Ankle Surg 2006;45(2):65–9.

79. Moore JA Jr, Shank JR, Morgan SJ, et al. Syndesmosis fixation: a comparison of three and four cortices of screw fixation without hardware removal. Foot Ankle Int 2006;27(8):567–72.

80. Hoiness P, Stromsoe K. Tricortical versus quadricortical syndesmosis fixation in ankle fractures: a prospective, randomized study comparing two methods of syndesmosis fixation. J Orthop Trauma 2004;18(6):331–7.

81. Thordarson DB, Samuelson M, Shepherd LE, et al. Bioabsorbable versus stainless steel screw fixation of the syndesmosis in pronation-lateral rotation ankle fractures: a prospective randomized trial. Foot Ankle Int 2001;22(4):335–8.

82. Hovis WD, Kaiser BW, Watson JT, et al. Treatment of syndesmotic disruptions of the ankle with bioabsorbable screw fixation. J Bone Joint Surg Am 2002;84-A(1):26–31.

83. Kaukonen JP, Lamberg T, Korkala O, et al. Fixation of syndesmotic ruptures in 38 patients with a malleolar fracture: a randomized study comparing a metallic and a bioabsorbable screw. J Orthop Trauma 2005;19(6):392–5.

84. Seitz WH Jr, Bachner EJ, Abram LJ, et al. Repair of the tibiofibular syndesmosis with a flexible implant. J Orthop Trauma 1991;5(1):78–82.

85. Thornes B, Walsh A, Hislop M, et al. Suture-endobutton fixation of ankle tibio-fibular diastasis: a cadaver study. Foot Ankle Int 2003;24(2):142–6.

86. Thornes B, Shannon F, Guiney AM, et al. Suture-button syndesmosis fixation: accelerated rehabilitation and improved outcomes. Clin Orthop Relat Res 2005; 431:207–12.

87. Kabukcuoglu Y, Kucukkaya M, Eren T, et al. The ANK device: a new approach in the treatment of the fractures of the lateral malleolus associated with the rupture of the syndesmosis. Foot Ankle Int 2000;21(9):753–8.

88. Jung HG, Nicholson JJ, Parks B, et al. Radiographic and biomechanical support for fibular plating of the agility total ankle. Clin Orthop Relat Res 2004;424: 118–24.

89. Espinosa N, Smerek JP, Myerson MS. Acute and chronic syndesmosis injuries: pathomechanisms, diagnosis and management. Foot Ankle Clin 2006;11(3): 639–57.

90. Henkemeyer U, Püschel R, Burri C. Experimentelle Untersuchungen zur Biome-
    chanik der Syndesmose. Annual Congress Supplement of Langenbeck's Archiv
    1975;369–71 [In German].
91. Rammelt S, Grass R, Zwipp H. Ankle fractures. Fuß and Sprunggelenk 2007;
    5(2):88–103 [in German].
92. Pottorff GT, Kaye RA. CT assessment of syndesmosis in Weber C ankle frac-
    tures. Paper presented at the American Orthopaedic Foot and Ankle Society
    Specialty Day, Washington DC, February 23, 1992.
93. Vasarhelyi A, Lubitz J, Gierer P, et al. Detection of fibular torsional deformities
    after surgery for ankle fractures with a novel CT method. Foot Ankle Int 2006;
    27(12):1115–21.
94. Ebraheim NA, Mekhail AO, Gargasz SS. Ankle fractures involving the fibula
    proximal to the distal tibiofibular syndesmosis. Foot Ankle Int 1997;18(8):513–21.
95. Kaye RA. Stabilization of ankle syndesmosis injuries with a syndesmosis screw.
    Foot Ankle 1989;9(6):290–3.
96. Chissell HR, Jones J. The influence of a diastasis screw on the outcome of
    Weber type-C ankle fractures. J Bone Joint Surg Br 1995;77(3):435–8.
97. Kennedy JG, Soffe KE, Dalla Vedova P, et al. Evaluation of the syndesmotic
    screw in low Weber C ankle fractures. J Orthop Trauma 2000;14(5):359–66.
98. Weening B, Bhandari M. Predictors of functional outcome following transsyndes-
    motic screw fixation of ankle fractures. J Orthop Trauma 2005;19(2):102–8.
99. McMaster JH, Scranton PE Jr. Tibiofibular synostosis: a cause of ankle disability.
    Clin Orthop Relat Res 1975;111:172–4.
100. Veltri DM, Pagnani MJ, O'Brien SJ, et al. Symptomatic ossification of the tibiofib-
    ular syndesmosis in professional football players: a sequela of the syndesmotic
    ankle sprain. Foot Ankle Int 1995;16(5):285–90.
101. Loder BG, Frascone ST, Wertheimer SJ. Tibiofibular arthrodesis for malunion of
    the talocrural joint. J Foot Ankle Surg 1995;34(3):283–8.
102. Ney R, Jend JJ, Schontag H. [Tibiofibular mobility and arthrosis in patients with
    postoperative ossification in the area of syndesmosis of the upper ankle joint].
    Unfallchirurgie 1987;13(5):274–7 [in German].
103. Mullins JF, Sallis JG. Recurrent sprain of the ankle joint with diastasis. J Bone
    Joint Surg Br 1958;40-B(2):270–3.
104. Castaing J, Le Chevallier PL, Meunier M. [Repeated sprain or recurring sublux-
    ation of the tibio-tarsal joint. A simple technic of external ligamentoplasty]. Rev
    Chir Orthop Reparatrice Appar Mot 1961;47:598–608 [in German].
105. Endres T, Grass R, Rammelt S, et al. Ankle arthrodesis with four cancellous lag
    screws. Oper Orthop Traumatol 2005;17(4–5):345–60.

Talus Fracture Management

John S. Early, MD[a,b,*]

KEYWORDS

- Talus fracture • Talar head fracture • Talar body fracture
- Talar neck fracture • Talar process fracture

The talus holds a key position in the normal locomotion of man. It is a vital part of both the ankle and subtalar complex of joints, which govern to a great degree the progression of normal gait. The bone itself is a small, irregularly shaped structure with no motor attachments and whose surface area is approximately 70% covered with articular cartilage. Vascular supply to the talus is fragile because of the limited extra-articular surface area available for intraosseous access. The extra-articular surface area serves also as an attachment site for the ligaments and joint capsules that provide the soft tissue stability to the tibiotalar and subtalar complex of joints. The shape of the talus controls both the motion and interaction of the ankle and subtalar complex joints. It is here that vertical weight-bearing forces are transferred into the horizontal support structures of the foot. Disruption of the normal bony contours can permanently impair both ankle motion and subtalar motion. Because of its importance, great care is needed in diagnosing and treating these injuries.

GENERAL CONSIDERATIONS

Fractures of the talus are many times easily missed, especially in the presence of other high-energy trauma. It is important to fully inspect and investigate any suspected injury as it is presented. The position of the foot on the body at rest can reveal a problem with talar positioning. Any resistance to subtalar or ankle motion should warrant radiographic investigation. When ordering radiographs, besides the routine ankle series, an anteroposterior (AP) view of the foot to fully view the talar head should also be obtained to be sure there are no secondary fractures that need to be addressed. I prefer to obtain a computed tomography (CT) scan of the talus with the minimal cut thickness available if any suspicion remains. It is better to conclusively rule out a fracture here than to miss it and have to perform reconstructive surgery later. Sagittal reconstruction slices also may be important in planning the surgical approach. These views will help determine the best approach for visualization, the optimal placement of fixation, and whether impaction of fragments will prevent reduction.

[a] Orthopaedic Surgery, University of Texas Southwestern Medical Center, Dallas, TX, USA
[b] Texas Orthopaedic Associates L.L.P, 8210 Walnut Hill Ln., Suite 130, Dallas, TX 75231, USA
* Texas Orthopaedic Associates L.L.P, 8210 Walnut Hill Ln., Suite 130, Dallas, TX 75231.
E-mail address: jearly@toaonline.com

Foot Ankle Clin N Am 13 (2008) 635–657
doi:10.1016/j.fcl.2008.08.005
1083-7515/08/$ – see front matter © 2008 Elsevier Inc. All rights reserved.

Postoperatively, patients with a talus fracture should remain non–weight bearing for at least 10 weeks. Rigid immobilization of the ankle and subtalar joint should be maintained for 6 weeks. The author recommends a well-molded cast with the ankle placed in full dorsiflexion and the hindfoot in neutral alignment. This appears to insure bony reduction of the talar dome and minimize anterior scar tissue formation. If a medial fixator is needed to maintain length or position of the head because of severe comminution, it should be left on for 6 to 8 weeks. At 6 weeks, gentle non–weight-bearing range of motion of both the subtalar and ankle joints should begin.[1–4] Exercise cycling appears to be a good way to work on motion and muscle conditioning without subjecting the foot to full weight bearing. Progressive weight bearing can then be instituted once the patient is comfortable.

Late complications such as arthritic pain and avascular necrosis are always a possibility with these fractures and should be discussed frequently with the patient.

FRACTURES OF THE TALAR HEAD

The literature on talar head fractures is sparse. In previously published series on talus fractures, less than 10% involve the talar head, either isolated or in concert with other talar injuries.[2,5–7] Information on treatment and long-term outcome for these rare fractures is not well documented. Most often, talar head fractures are found in conjunction with other fractures resulting from a high-energy impact, both of the talus and adjacent structures.

Talar head fractures can occur along the talonavicular joint proper and in the middle facet. They are the result of a compressive load delivered either through the sustentaculum of the calcaneus and or the navicular with an axial load. Various investigators feel that dorsiflexion and inversion of the foot is the mechanism of injury producing the fracture pattern. This loading can result in two distinct fracture patterns, a crush injury to the articular surface with significant comminution or a shear fracture **(Fig. 1)**.[2] The articular crush injury is seen most often at the middle facet area of the talar head and can result in significant damage to the plantar talar head. It often is the area missed initially because it is so difficult to visualize radiographically. Impaction of sustentaculum into the talar head without reduction will completely eliminate motion in the subtalar joint and create a mild varus heel position. A crush injury to the talar head via the navicular can also occur with significant destruction of the joint surface. The presence of a displaced shear fracture most often occurs medially and indicates that there was a partial uncovering of the affected joint surface by inversion of the foot before the axial load. These fractures can be seen in isolation but more often are found in the presence of subtalar subluxation or dislocation. Talar head injuries also can be associated with a lateral column injury most likely involving a fracture of the cuboid. For this reason, it is important to rule out a talar head injury any time a patient presents with a subtalar or talonavicular dislocation. It is not uncommon for a medial subtalar complex dislocation to have a medial talar shear fracture. This displacement will cause medial column shortening and act as a block to subtalar joint reduction **(Fig. 2)**.

Diagnostic evaluation of a suspected talar head injury includes a simple AP radiograph of the foot, which should be obtained with every ankle injury to preliminarily assess the talonavicular joint. The crush component to the middle facet is more difficult visualize and usually requires a CT scan. A CT scan is therefore indicated in the event of any talar head injury.

Actual series reports on the treatment and results of these fractures are limited. The goals of treatment are to restore normal subtalar complex motion and maintain the

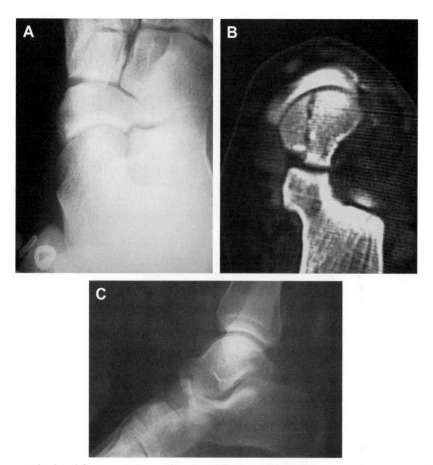

Fig. 1. Talar head fracture patterns. (*A, B*) Simple shear fracture. (*C, D*) Shear fracture with nonreducible medial subluxation of talonavicular joint. (*E, F*) Shear fracture with middle facet comminution and impaction.

weight-bearing architecture of the talus. For the crush injury to the middle facet of the talar head caused by the sustentaculum, treatment should depend on the observed mobility of the subtalar joint once all other injuries to the foot are stable. If there is an impaction of the middle facet significant enough to block motion of the sustentaculum across the plantar surface of the talar head, an attempt should be made to restore the plantar head contour. This is necessary to allow smooth gliding motion of the sustentaculum, which occurs with movement of the posterior facet. If, in the treatment of adjacent injuries, the area is exposed and there is no evidence of joint restriction, any loose fragments present in the joint should be removed. There is no literature to suggest that anatomic restoration of the plantar joint surface offers any long-term advantage once motion is restored. Long-term effects of this fracture are not known.

The surgical approach for the middle facet injury is an incision between the tibialis anterior and tibialis posterior tendons extending from the medial malleolus to the navicular tubercle. After a longitudinal incision into the talonavicular joint capsule, the crush injury can be visualized, and debridement or elevation can be performed. In the event of a plantar impaction injury, a cortical window can be created

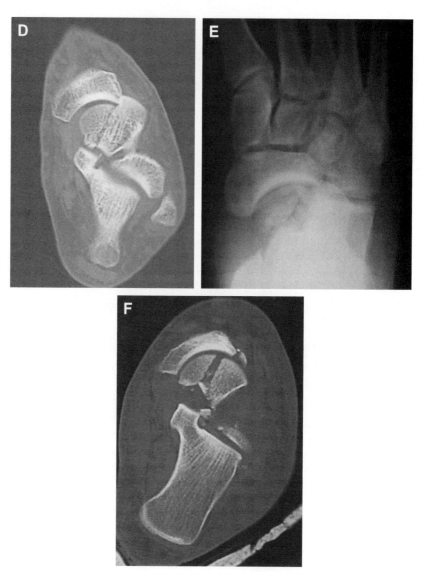

Fig. 1. (*continued*)

dorsomedially in the talar neck, through which a bone tamp is used to disimpact the plantar cortex. The articular reduction is assessed by watching the sustentaculum glide over the area. Once reduction is satisfactory, bone graft is placed behind the surgically created defect for support. My personal preference with these rare injuries is to use a cannulated reamer to create the hole down to within 1 cm of the impaction area, saving the reamings for later use. After restoring the articular surface, bone graft substitute is formed into a cylinder and has some resistance to compression. The appropriate cylinder is tamped into place and covered with graft dorsally to add resistance to settling. With this technique, fixation usually is not needed. If there is a shear fracture of the medial head in addition to the impaction, a direct approach to the impaction

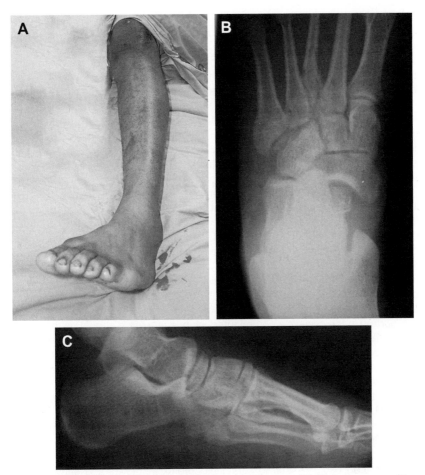

Fig. 2. Fixed talonavicular subluxation with talar head fracture. (*A*) Clinical varus position of foot with locked talonavicular joint. (*B, C*) Radiographs show bony overlap at talonavicular joint.

can be performed, and the fixation of the medial shear fragment will act as the support for the weight-bearing surface. Mini-fragment screws or bioabsorbable screws can be used for fixation. My preference in this instance is to use bioabsorbable implants.

Fractures to the talonavicular portion of the talar head are treated based on the integrity of the medial column as well as the stability of the joint. A stable, reduced joint, with a nondisplaced fracture can be treated nonoperatively as long as the fragment does not shift with motion through the talonavicular joint, and the joint itself is stable. This can be studied two ways. One is with the use of fluoroscopic imaging while moving the talonavicular joint. The second method is using plain AP radiographs with the foot fully inverted and then fully everted. Both methods will indicate whether the joint and fragment are stable. The majority of displaced talar head fractures are unstable. Free-floating fragments or any interruption in the smooth motion of the talonavicular joint should be addressed surgically in an attempt to limit long-term degeneration. A crush injury to the talar head usually causes severe comminution of the articular surface and shortening of the talar neck. This shortening causes an imbalance between the medial and lateral columns of the foot. In treating this injury, restoration of normal medial column length is of primary importance closely followed by restoration of articular contour.

The approach to the shear component of a talar head fracture is felt by some to be best accessed through a medial approach.[2,7] In the author's experience, this is only effective if the fragment lies on the medial side of the talar head, and sufficient dissection of the capsule is done to adequately visualize the articular fracture line. I prefer a dorsal longitudinal incision directly over the fracture extending beyond the talonavicular joint, which offers the best visualization for reduction of the displaced articular surface while requiring minimal dissection. This approach is extremely important in those cases involving fixed subluxation of the talonavicular joint because of the articular stepoff (**Fig. 3**). During the exposure, great care is taken not to dissect the capsule off the talar neck. Subperiosteal dissection over the dorsum of the navicular usually will allow adequate visualization of the joint surface. In the case of Chopart joint instability or difficult visualization, a small external fixator is used to distract the joint for visualization. The fixation pins are placed medially with distal pins in the cuneiform and or navicular. Proximal pins can be placed in the talar neck, medial malleolus, or calcaneal sustentaculum.

Simple fractures can be fixed using k-wires, mini fragment screws, or bioabsorbable implants. With a medial exposure, the implants are placed under direct visualization. With the dorsal approach, fixation is placed percutaneously from either the medial or lateral cortex. In the case of a comminuted injury every effort should be made to preserve the talonavicular joint. Free floating cartilage fragments should be removed. The impacted or comminuted head can be molded against the navicular contour. This is best done with the talonavicular joint in a neutral position and held by a medial placed external fixator. Bone graft is usually required to fill in the void created by the restoration of the talar neck length and can be obtained from the calcaneus, distal tibia, or proximal tibia. Fragments too small for fixation or free floating should be excised.

The incidence of posttraumatic arthritis and the value of operative repair are not discussed in the literature. In the author's experience, severe comminution of the talar head will lead to early talonavicular arthritis. Those injuries not recognized as unstable or left untreated usually result in subtalar complex instability and early arthritis. In those fractures treated operatively, either with debridement or early stabilization, no trend toward early arthritis has been seen.

TALAR NECK FRACTURES

Talar neck fractures occur through the extra-articular portion of the talus and represent almost 50% of all talus fractures.[1,4,7,8] The mechanism of injury is usually described by a combination of forced ankle dorsiflexion followed by axial compression of the tibiotalar joint. Because of the early recognition and extensive literature on this type of fracture, there are a number of radiographic views described to visualize the neck. In the author's opinion, a CT scan is more effective at giving the surgeon a complete picture of the injury as well as information on the surrounding structures.[9] Although there have been volumes written on the classification schemes and complications inherent with these injuries, recent literature shows that early, anatomic restoration of anatomy with rigid fixation offers the surgeon the best chance of a good result.[10,11]

The literature is replete with the debate on open versus closed treatment for these fractures and the implants best suited for the purpose. The only neck fracture that should be treated without surgery is a true type 1 fracture which is rare and usually

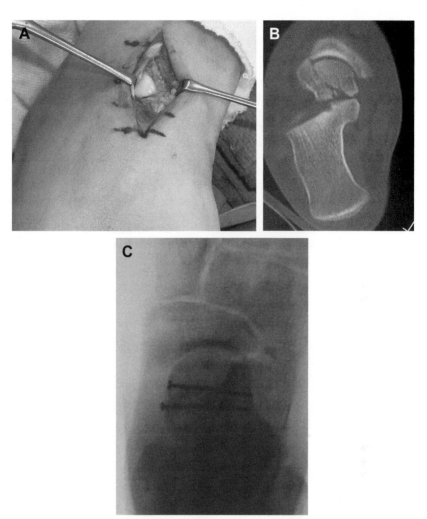

Fig. 3. Surgical approach to the talar head. (*A*) Dorsal approach shows talar head fracture with medial dislocation of navicular. This approach allows direct visualization of fracture and joint reduction. Fixation is percutaneously placed. (*B*) CT scan of fracture anatomy. (*C*) Postoperative radiograph shows screw placement through percutaneous introduction from the medial side. Seating of the heads onto bone can be directly visualized through the dorsal incision.

only recognized as an incidental finding on a CT scan. The treatment is rigid immobilization and non–weight bearing for 6 to 8 weeks as described earlier.

Any fracture visualized on plain radiographs has to have had some degree of displacement or the fracture density would not change; however, it is the rotational malalignment component that typically allows an otherwise seemingly nondisplaced fracture to be visible. It is important to easily visualize the fracture in multiple planes so that true anatomic reduction in all planes can be achieved. It is also important to open the fracture to remove incarcerated fragments; any loose debris that may be in the subtalar joint is only accessible when the fracture is distracted. My preferred approach is to use two incisions, a medial and anterior lateral.

The medial approach begins on the anterior border of the medial malleolus and bisects the space between the tibialis anterior and posterior tendons. The incision is curved proximally along the axis of the tibia to allow visualization of tibiotalar joint.

The anterior lateral incision follows the extensor digitorum bundle from the tibiotalar joint to the lateral border of the navicular and lateral cuneiform bones. The extensor retinaculum is transected in a "Z" fashion to allow subsequent closure. With the extensor tendons laterally displaced, direct visualization of the lateral dome of the talar head, the shoulder of the neck and body and the neck are possible. Distraction of the tibiotalar joint can be done if reduction of the body is necessary. Sometimes a large Schanz pin is used to grab the body through the exposed neck fracture to pull it back to its reduced position. Rotational realignment of the head onto the body is done with direct visualization.

Fixation will depend on the extent and location of comminution—it is always easiest to reduce and pin the least comminuted side first to gauge the position of true reduction. With the limited space for fixation, especially on the medial side, the author recommends using guide wires for cannulated screws as a means of temporary fixation and a potential guide for permanent stability. Bone grafting may be necessary to fill in any defect on the comminuted side to provide support for the desired neck position (**Fig. 4**).

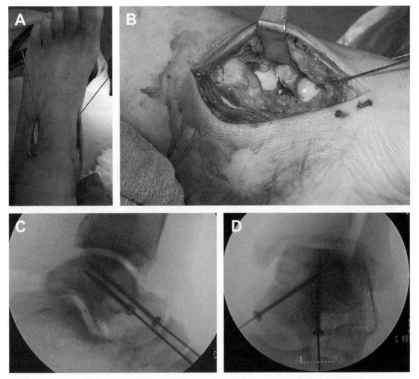

Fig. 4. Surgical approach to talar neck fractures. (*A*) Intraoperative picture of surgical incisions to visualize neck. (*B*) medial view of reduction along medial facet of talus. Guide wire in talar head. (*C, D*) Intraoperative radiographs of fixation position for simple neck fracture.

Once the bone is reduced and stable at the fracture site, the method of fixation can be determined.[12] In simple minimally comminuted fracture patterns, cannulated screws appear easiest. They can be introduced in a variety of places, though I find the posterior approach advocated by some as too difficult with the use of anterior visualization. Screw fixation can go through the talonavicular cartilage surface if necessary as long as the screw heads are sufficiently buried that they do not come into contact with navicular cartilage. Mini fragment plates are preferred in the event of significant comminution and act as bridge plates to stabilize the two sides and the intervening graft. Once optimal reduction and fixation has been obtained, subtalar motion is assessed to ensure against impinging implants or bony malalignment obstructing full motion.

TALAR BODY FRACTURES

Talar body fractures, though more common than talar head fractures, account for only 7% to 38% of all fractures of the talus.[1,4,7,8] A recent review from a major trauma canter found the overall percentage of talar body injuries when compared with all fractures treated was 0.62%. Furthermore, talar body injuries were seen in only 6.8% of patients with specific foot injuries and in only 24% of all talar injuries.[1] The majority of injuries to the talus primarily involve the talar neck. To distinguish between neck and body fractures, talar body fractures are now defined to include all injuries to the talus that produce a fracture line at or posterior to the lateral tubercle of the talus.[13] For the purpose of discussion, these fractures will be divided into the body proper involving the central dome of the tibial talar joint, including the traumatic osteochondral fracture, and peripheral fractures of the lateral process, posterior medial, and posterior lateral tubercles. These peripheral fractures involve mainly the posterior facet of the subtalar joint complex.

The shear fracture of the talar body often is referred to as an acute osteochondral fracture because of the thin bone fragment attached to the overlying cartilage. Typically, these injuries are seen in gymnasts, cheerleaders, and other athletes who perform maneuvers in the air and are then required to land on the ground standing. These can present as severe ankle sprains associated with painful weight bearing. Any patient presenting with this scenario should undergo plain radiographic evaluation and will likely require a CT to fully delineate the pathology (**Fig. 5**). The majority occur on the lateral dome. The fragment usually is found inverted with the bony surface exposed to the tibia and incarcerated in the joint, and therefore requires urgent attention.

The fracture is approached through the side most accessible to the talar defect, which can be medial or lateral. In most cases, an osteotomy is not needed. Lateral injuries usually are aided by the fact that the anterior talo-fibular ligament is disrupted. Arthroscopic attempts to treat this injury with anything other than fragment debridement are very difficult because the fragment is flipped, and there is little room and few instruments available to turn the piece over while enclosed in the joint.

Once the fracture fragment is retrieved from the joint and the talar defect visualized, the surgeon must decide to either discard or stabilize the fracture fragment; if the fragment has attached bone and is big enough to accept fixation, stabilization with bioabsorbable pins should be attempted in the acute setting. If the fragment is deemed too small or appropriate fixation is not available, the fragment should be discarded and the defect treated similar to an arthroscopic osteochondral debridement.

A fracture of the talar body proper is secondary to high-energy trauma and rarely seen in isolation.[1] The major force is axial loading with the variation in the fracture pattern caused in part by variable foot positioning at the time of loading. The patterns

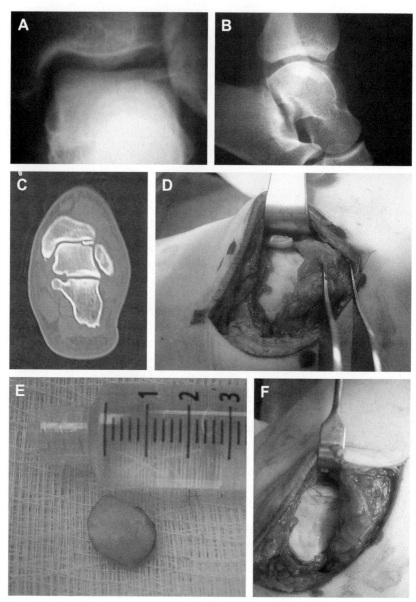

Fig. 5. Acute osteochondral fracture of talus. (*A–C*) Injury films of lateral talar injury. CT shows incarceration of fragment in joint. (*D*) Initial exposure of fracture through disrupted lateral ligaments show inversion of fragment. (*E*) actual fragment after debridement of fibrous tissue. (*F*) Intraoperative view of reattached fragment on talus. A bioabsorbable barbed tack was used for fixation.

vary from simple two-part fractures to multifragmented injuries with significant articular destruction (**Fig. 6**). It is important to realize that body fractures involve both the subtalar and tibiotalar joint. The literature describes attempts to classify the various body fracture patterns, but to date these classification schemas have not been shown to have any significance for either treatment choices or outcome.[1,4,11,14,15]

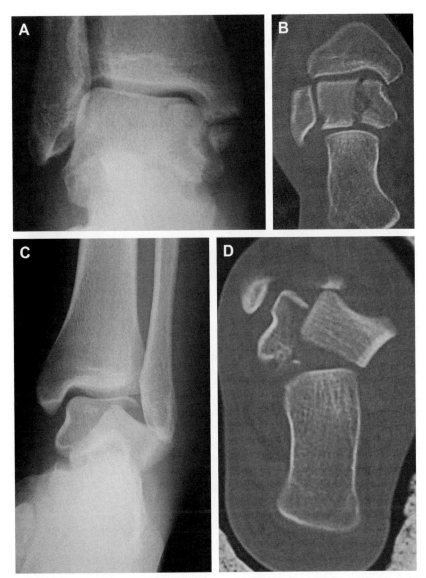

Fig. 6. Talar body fracture patterns. (*A, B*) Sagittal plane fracture of the talar dome. (*C, D*) Frontal plane fracture of the talar dome. (*E, F*) Comminuted fracture of the talar dome.

Treatment of talar body fractures is based on restoring joint integrity of both the tibiotalar and subtalar joints.[1,2,7,11,16] Despite high rates of posttraumatic arthritis in both the ankle and subtalar joints, the consensus opinion is that all talar body fractures should be treated with anatomic reduction and internal fixation. Even in the case of severe comminution, every attempt should be made to restore at least the tibiotalar articulation once the soft tissues have settled enough to permit surgery. The use of internal fixation over k-wire fixation will allow earlier motion, and commonly used implants include mini fragment screws and bioabsorbable tacks. These fractures involve articular fragments with little or no extra articular surface area.

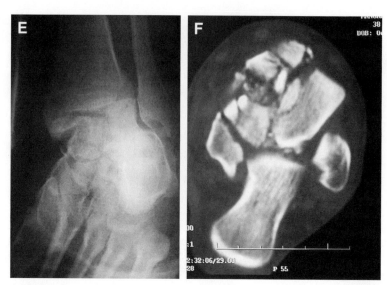

Fig. 6. (*continued*)

The open reduction of talar body fractures should be performed through a two-incision approach:[1–3,11] one incision should be based medially and the second laterally just along the anterior border of the fibula. Access to the tibiotalar and subtalar joint surfaces should be possible from either incision, and an osteotomy of either malleolus can be performed where needed to affect reduction or fixation. Although not every talar body fracture requires a malleolar osteotomy for visualization or fixation, it is important to be prepared to perform one if it is needed during the surgery. A preoperative CT scan will greatly assist in deciding if one is needed.

An osteotomy of the tibia is performed more often over the more comminuted side of the talar body side to allow direct access to the fracture fragments. It is important when creating an osteotomy to make it of sufficient size to allow easy visualization of the dome fragments. To access the medial talar dome, a large oblique osteotomy of the tibial plafond is preferred to gain unfettered visualization of the joint surface. I believe it is best to make the osteotomy enter the joint past the injured portion of the talus to avoid having any disruption of the plafond over the healing fracture. Once created, the medial fragment is reflected distally on the deltoid attachment, which requires release of the anterior capsule and posterior tibialis retinaculum. Once work on the talus is completed, the osteotomy is best fixed with a simple five-hole one-third tubular plate and 3.5-mm screws to provide compression of the osteotomy site and prevent any dorsal migration of the medial fragment (**Fig. 7**).

Lateral dome access is more difficult—the key is not to limit visualization of the damaged talar surface. The best method is to again take a generous portion of the overlying plafond in an oblique manner. If the area is limited to the anterior lateral portion, a large double-cut osteotomy of the Chaput tubercle of the tibia can be performed, leaving the syndesmosis intact (**Fig. 8**). For more exposure, both a fibular osteotomy and a lateral plafond osteotomy may be needed to gain working access to the fracture, which again allows maintenance of the syndesmosis ligaments. Fixation of this osteotomy will require plating of both the tibia and fibula to hold the reduction. If only posterior medial comminution is noted, access similar to that described for posterior medial tubercle fractures can be used without the need for osteotomies. These issues illustrate the

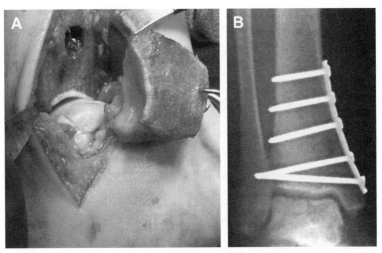

Fig. 7. Medial tibial osteotomy for talar access. (*A*) Large medial tibial osteotomy for direct visualization of talar dome surface. (*B*) Postoperative fixation with plate to prevent migration.

importance of a preoperative CT scan of the talus to allow proper planning of the approaches necessary to maximize reduction of the joint surface.

The first step in reconstructing the talar dome should be to disengage all the fragments so that the subtalar joint can be visualized if injured and cleared of debris. Any impacted surfaces should be elevated and grafted if necessary. Graft is easily obtained from the tibia, especially if an osteotomy is used to access the talus. Impacted surfaces on the subtalar side are addressed first because they will be inaccessible once the dome is reassembled. The fracture fragments should then be reduced and pinned into place. Intercalary fragments should be reduced and pinned to one of the outer surfaces before fixing the two sides together. Only when the body is

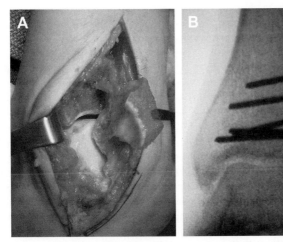

Fig. 8. Lateral tibial osteotomy for talus access. (*A*) Chaput fragment rotated out on syndesmosis ligaments to visualize lateral dome fracture. (*B*) Postoperative fixation of osteotomy site. Bioabsorbable implants were used to stabilize talus.

completely reassembled should permanent fixation be implanted. All definitive implants should lie in either the medial or lateral gutter. Bioabsorbable tacks or compression screws are preferable if fixation is needed on the weight-bearing dome. Otherwise, mini fragment titanium screws should be considered over stainless steel if possible, to facilitate future magnetic resonance imaging evaluation if needed.

LATERAL PROCESS FRACTURES

The lateral process fracture of the talus is frequently referred to as a "snow boarder's fracture" because of its frequency of appearance in snowboarders with ankle injuries. It is also the second most common of fracture of the talar body.[17] Up to 24% of all talar body injuries involve the lateral process.[2] Its reported incidence is as high as 15% of all ankle injuries and 34% of ankle fractures in one series.[18] The mechanism of injury requires the foot to be in a dorsiflexed and inverted position.[17] This rotation of the posterior talocalcaneal facet uncovers the lateral process. Axial compression then produces asymmetric loading of the process between the fibula and the calcaneus. The fragment usually includes the attachment of the talocalcaneal and anterior talofibular ligaments. The fracture fragment can be variable in size and often is minimally displaced. In those resulting from motor vehicle or high-energy impact trauma, significant damage can occur to the subtalar joint.

The major difficulty with lateral process fractures is the frequency with which they are missed.[3,17,19-23] Often they are found as the result of chronic pain for an ankle sprain. In the case of an isolated injury, it is important to carefully examine any patient presenting with an ankle sprain and a history of impact loading. Lateral process fractures are point tender in the sinus tarsi where the process is palpable.[2,19] Careful scrutiny of mortise and lateral radiographs is necessary to visualize the fracture, yet nondisplaced fractures can still easily be missed (**Fig. 9**). CT evaluation of the talus should thus be completed whenever a lateral process injury is suspected.[2,18] Fracture fragment displacement and the extent of articular involvement are best assessed on coronal CT scan (1.5 mm cuts throughout the talus) (**Fig. 10**).

Treatment depends on the presence of intra-articular displacement of the fragment or fragments.[3,21-23] A nondisplaced injury to the lateral process can be treated in a non–weight-bearing cast for 4 to 6 weeks;[18] weight bearing then can be advanced as comfort allows. Nonoperative treatment of displaced fractures has led to uniformly poor results.[19,24,25] Displaced fractures should therefore be managed with open anatomic reduction and fixation or debridement. Every effort should be made to restore the articular congruity of the subtalar joint; only if the fragments are too small for secure fixation should they be excised from the joint.[3,21]

The surgical approach to the lateral process is through the sinus tarsi (**Fig. 11**). A curvilinear incision from the midpoint of the lateral malleolus to the calcaneal cuboid joint is used. The incision goes from just superior to the tip of the lateral malleolus, directly over the lateral process, and along the floor of the sinus tarsi. The extensor brevis muscle should not be disturbed. The subtalar joint capsule should be opened, and the subtalar joint visually inspected. It is here where the loose fragments of the impacted joint surface are identified. It is important to recognize and reduce any impaction of the subtalar joint before stabilizing the external articular fragments. Fixation of suitable fractures can be accomplished with bioabsorbable screws or mini fragment (1.5 mm–2.7 m) screws and plates. The actual implant configuration depends on the fracture. Fracture fragment debridement should be done only when the fragments are too small to support fixation, and in this instance all intra-articular debris must be removed to reduce the incidence of arthritis.

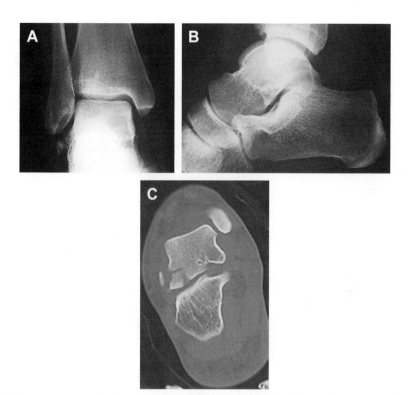

Fig. 9. Lateral process fractures of the talus. (*A, B*) Typical radiographic presentation of lateral process fracture. (*C*) CT scan highlights subtalar involvement.

Postoperatively, the foot is placed into a non–weight-bearing cast for 6 weeks, followed by progressive range of motion and weight bearing as comfort allows. The greatest complication occurs with missing this fracture.[3,21] Closed treatment of displaced fractures or early weight bearing of nondisplaced injuries can lead to subtalar arthritis. The results of anatomic stabilization do not appear to have high subtalar arthritis rates.[4,19,26]

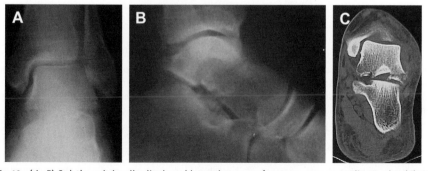

Fig. 10. (*A, B*) Subtle, minimally displaced lateral process fracture seen on radiographs. (*C*) CT scan shows significant impaction to subtalar surface in addition to minimally displaced fracture.

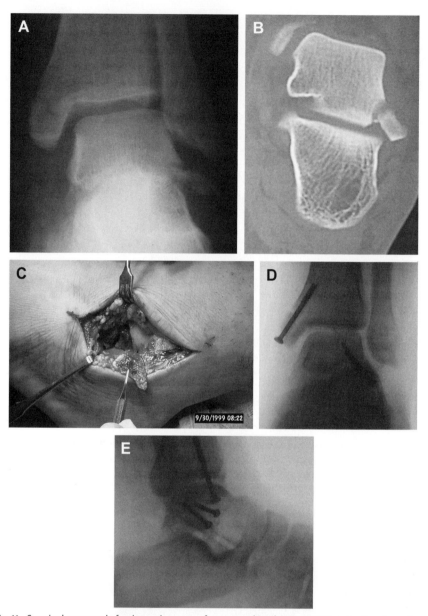

Fig. 11. Surgical approach for lateral process fractures. (*A, B*) Preoperative studies show fracture pattern. (*C*) Intraoperative view of surgical approach. The fracture fragment is rotated outward to show posterior facet of calcaneus and inspect the subtalar joint. (*D, E*) Postoperative films.

POSTERIOR MEDIAL TALUS FRACTURES

Fractures of the posterior aspect of the talus also are seen and reported separately from true body fractures. They can involve the lateral tubercle, os trigonum, or the medial tubercle. The os trigonum fracture is more common and is caused by hyper plantar flexion loads. Fracture of the posterior medial aspect of the talar body is the rarest of reported talar injuries. They exist as case reports in the literature for both operative and nonoperative care.[4,27–33]

The inferior surface of the medial tubercle is part of the posterior facet of the subtalar joint; the extra-articular portion provides an attachment for the posterior tibiotalar ligament, and its dorsal surface is involved with the tibiotalar joint. There are two described mechanisms for producing this injury: it may occur by a direct blow to the area directly behind the medial malleolus or be the result of a pronation, dorsiflexion load to the posterior medial talus.[28,34] It is described as the result of sports, fall from heights, and motor vehicle collisions.[4,27–33]

The greatest problem with this injury, like others in the talus, is recognition.[2,31,32] Even with multiple radiographic images, this type of injury can be difficult to see (**Fig. 12**). Pain or fullness posterior to the medial malleolus from trauma warrants a high index of suspicion for posterior medial talar injury. Further workup should include a fine-cut (1.5 mm) CT scan of the talus, which shows not only the fracture but also the extent of involvement of the subtalar and tibiotalar joints. Failure to recognize and treat this injury appears to uniformly lead to subtalar arthritis and fusion. Displaced fragments can also impinge on posterior tibialis function or create posterior tibial nerve pressure. Current recommendations call for aggressive management, including open reduction and internal fixation of displaced fractures. There are no reports of recognized, nondisplaced posterior medial fractures. Therefore, the effect of nonoperative treatment on these injuries is not known. Displaced fractures treated with immobilization have a uniformly poor outcome leading to subtalar fusion.[35,36]

The operative approach to this injury is from the medial side of the ankle.[28,35] If the fracture does not extend distal to the posterior one third of the medial aspect of the talar body, the whole fracture should then lie directly behind the medial malleolus, particularly with dorsiflexion of the ankle (**Fig. 13**). This is an important distinction that can be seen on CT scan. The need for a medial malleolar osteotomy will dictate the position of the skin incision; the majority of posterior medial talar fractures will not require a medial malleolar osteotomy, and, in these instances, creating an osteotomy can actually impair visualization of the posterior talus. The best visualization is through a curvilinear approach parallel to the posterior tibial tendon. The tendon sheath is incised carefully to allow later repair, and the tendon is displaced over the medial malleolus and covered by a moist cloth. The posterior capsule is then excised off the tibial attachment from the tip of the malleolus to the syndesmosis. The capsule and flexor digitorum longus tendon is retracted posteriorly. This will allow visualization of the posterior aspect of the talus, the tibiotalar joint, and the subtalar joint. Dorsiflexion of the ankle will facilitate visualization of any dome extension of the fracture for reconstruction.

Anatomic reduction is best achieved by first separating the fracture fragments. The joint surfaces then are assessed for chondral injury or subchondral impaction. The deep surfaces are reconstructed first, followed by the subtalar surface, and finally the tibiotalar surface. Many times cancellous graft is needed to fill the void between the two joint surfaces and give some stiffness to the repair. Mini fragment screws and or bioabsorbable implants are used to secure fragments. Both the tibiotalar and subtalar joints should be passively ranged before closure to ensure against stepoff or impingement of articular surfaces.

Os trigonum injuries sometimes are hard to distinguish from contusion. The pain generated is directly behind the tibia. Palpable tenderness is found in the soft tissues behind the Achilles tendon and usually does not involve the peroneal or posterior tibialis tendons. Again, a CT scan should be obtained for initial evaluation. If suspected, simple

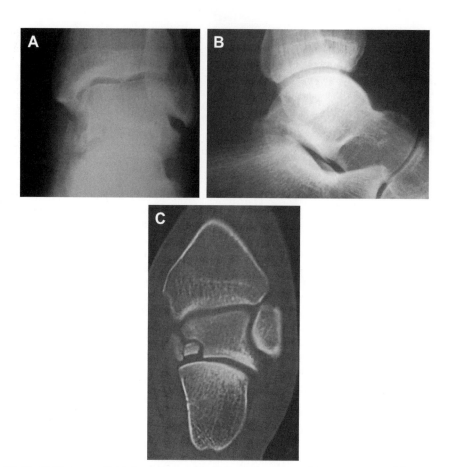

Fig. 12. Posterior medial talar fracture. (*A, B*) Typical radiographic appearance of fracture. (*C*) CT scan shows extent of subtalar and tibiotalar injury.

immobilization for 6 weeks typically will lead to full resolution of symptoms; however, the majority of these injuries are recognized only later when continued posterior ankle pain is present with activity. Optimal treatment consists of complete excision through a posterior–lateral approach. The incision is made just behind the fibula while avoiding the sural nerve. The peroneal retinaculum is not disturbed, but the posterior aspect of the tibia is located deep and followed to the lateral tubercle. With direct visualization of the talar and subtalar joints, the bony fragments are removed. The flexor hallucis longus tendon lies just beyond these fragments and can be injured if the associated soft tissue attachments are not sufficiently released as the fragment is removed.

For the acute fracture, rigid immobilization and restricted weight bearing still is the preferred treatment. After surgical excision, however, weight bearing can begin immediately, although I still prefer rigid immobilization to allow sufficient time for the disrupted posterior ligaments to heal.

OPEN FRACTURES

Fractures of the talus with open wounds present challenges more so to the issue of wound and soft tissue management rather than the actual fracture management.

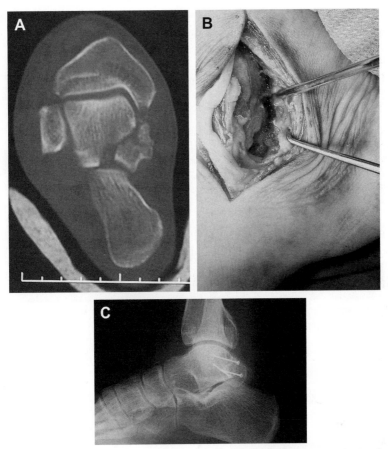

Fig. 13. Surgical approach to posterior medial fractures. (*A*) preoperative CT depicts fracture pattern. Note that the fracture is inferior and posterior to the medial malleolus. An osteotomy to view this fracture would actually hinder access. (*B*) Intraoperative view of approach. The posterior tibialis is dislocated anteriorly over the medial malleolus, and the posterior medial capsule to the talus is elevated off the talus. With dorsiflexion of the ankle, the talar dome is brought into the wound. (*C*) Immediate postoperative fixation.

Fracture reduction should be attempted through the cleaned wound, if possible, and at the time of planned wound closure, because this may represent the most optimal opportunity for an anatomic reduction. Even if a free flap is needed to provide coverage, fracture fixation should be attempted before the wound is sealed to maximize potential recovery. A dead or malunited talus with scarred, compromised tissue is a difficult problem to correct. Acute dislocation of the body or head or neck should be reduced emergently because these represent a significant threat to the surrounding soft tissues, causing pressure necrosis if left unattended. Fixation techniques for the potential components do not differ from those described above.

CRUSH FRACTURES

High-load injuries usually cause multiple fracture lines, which can encompass the entire talus. These injuries are severe and usually lead to significant complications

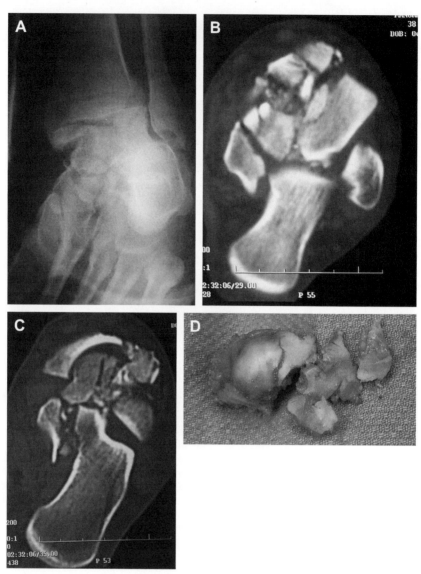

Fig. 14. Severe talar injury. (*A–C*) Preoperative studies depict crush injury of both the talar body and head. In this case, the subtalar and talonavicular joints could not be salvaged. (*D*) Intraoperative picture of comminution of talar head and subtalar joint surfaces. (*E–G*) Immediate postoperative views of reconstruction of the tibiotalar joint in addition to an acute fusion of the subtalar and talonavicular joints. (*G, H*) Four-year follow-up of case. No ankle pain with full activity.

involving both the ankle and subtalar complex joints. There are advocates for both immediate fusion as well as staged external fixation and delayed fusion.[2] Other investigators prefer at least an attempt at joint salvage with open reduction and internal fixation. The choice actually is governed by the damage to the soft tissue envelope. Open wounds, severe edema, and abrasions all will lead to compromise of the ideal

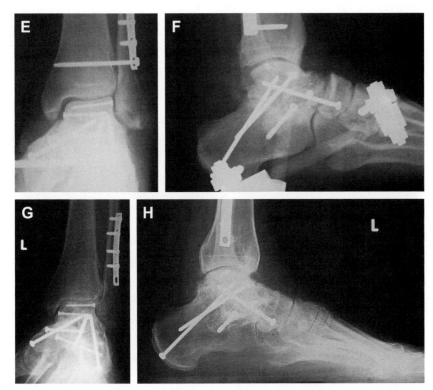

Fig. 14. (*continued*)

goal for internal reconstruction and fixation. Sometimes the fragmentation of the bone leaves little to reconstruct. In any event, when the skin permits, every effort should be made to restore at least the tibiotalar joint surface. Next in importance is restoring the length of the medial column and providing a strong support for the navicular. If reconstruction of the subtalar and talonavicular joints is possible, it should be attempted. If not, an acute fusion of that joint in a reduced position should be done to preserve foot position (**Fig. 14**). Only as a last resort should consideration be given to a pantalar fusion. This option is reserved for severe comminution when even the tibiotalar joint surface is not salvageable.[7]

There is always a role for attempting to salvage the tibiotalar joint in a severely comminuted talus fracture. This may require sacrifice or acute fusion of the subtalar and or the talonavicular joints to secure foot position and maintain some ankle motion. This can be successful if attempted as soon as the soft tissues will allow. The approach is governed by the pattern of the fracture at the dome and obtaining an anatomic reduction of that surface. Structural bone graft may be needed to restore position of the foot under the dome.

SUMMARY

Talar head and body injuries are not easily recognized and can create significant long-term disability when missed. Careful investigation of any injury about the ankle requires both clinical and radiographic examination. A CT scan is extremely helpful in diagnosing and treating these injuries. Displaced fractures require open reduction of the major joint surfaces and internal fixation. Prolonged non-weight bearing and immobilization is the norm. And despite aggressive management, complications involving avascular necrosis, and posttraumatic arthritis to both the subtalar and ankle joints occurs frequently.

REFERENCES

1. Vallier HA, Nork SE, Benirschke SK, et al. Surgical treatment of talar body fractures. J Bone Joint Surg Am 2003;85-A(9):1716–24.
2. Sanders R. Fractures and fracture-dislocations of the talus [chapter 35]. In: Coughlin M, Mann R, editors. Surgery of the foot and ankle. St Louis (MO): Mosby; 1999. p. 1465–518.
3. Heckman JD. Fractures of the talus [chapter 48]. In: Bucholz RW, Heckman JD, editors. Fractures in adults. Philadelphia: Lippincott; 2001.
4. Elgafy H, Ebraheim NA, Tile M, et al. Fractures of the talus: experience of two level 1 trauma centers. Foot Ankle Int 2000;21(12):1023–9.
5. Canale S, Kelly F. Fractures of the neck of the talus. Long term evaluation of seventy-one cases. J Bone Joint Surg Am 1978;60(2):143–56.
6. Adelaar RS. The treatment of complex fractures of the talus. Orthop Clin North Am 1989;20(4):691–707.
7. Adelaar RS. Complex fractures of the talus [chapter 7]. In: Adelaar RS, editor. Complex foot and ankle trauma. Philadelphia: Lippincott-Raven; 1999. p. 65–94.
8. Higgins T, Baumgaertner M. Diagnosis and treatment of fractures of the talus: a comprehensive review of the literature. Foot Ankle Int 1999;20(9):595–605.
9. Chan G, Sanders DW, Yuan X, et al. Clinical accuracy of imaging techniques for talar neck malunion. J Orthop Trauma 2008;22(6):415–8.
10. Vallier HA, Nork SE, Barei DP, et al. Talar neck fractures: results and outcomes. J Bone Joint Surg Am 2004;86-A(8):1616–24.
11. Lindvall E, Haidukewych G, DiPasquale T, et al. Open reduction and stable fixation of isolated, displaced talar neck and body fractures. J Bone Joint Surg Am 2004;86-A(10):2229–34.
12. Attiah M, Sanders DW, Valdivia G, et al. Comminuted talar neck fractures: a mechanical comparison of fixation techniques. J Orthop Trauma 2007;21(1):47–51.
13. Inokuchi S, Ogawa K, Usami N. Classification of fractures of the talus: clear differentiation between neck and body fractures. Foot Ankle Int 1996;17:748–50.
14. Fortin P, Balazsy J. Talus fractures: evaluation and treatment. J Am Acad Orthop Surg 2001;9:114–27.
15. Frawley P, Hart J, Young D. Treatment outcome of major fractures of the talus. Foot Ankle Int 1995;16(6):339–45.
16. Grob D, Simpson LA, Weber BG, et al. Operative treatment of displaced talus fractures. Clin Orthop Relat Res 1985;199:88–96.
17. Hawkins LG. Fracture of the lateral process of the talus. J Bone Joint Surg Am 1965;47:1170–5.
18. Kirkpatrick DP, Hunter RE, Janes PC, et al. The Snowboarder's foot and ankle. Am J Sports Med 1998;26(2):271–7.
19. Mukherjee SK, Pringle RM, Baxter AD. Fracture of the lateral process of the talus. A report of thirteen cases. J Bone Joint Surg Br 1974;56(2):263–73.
20. Thordarson DB. Talar body fractures. Orthop Clin North Am 2001;32(1):65–77.
21. Heckman JD, McLean MR. Fractures of the lateral process of the talus. Clin Orthop Relat Res 1985;(199):108–13.

22. von Knoch F, Reckord F, von Knoch M, et al. Fracture of the lateral process of the talus in snowboarders. J Bone Joint Surg Br 2007;89(6):772–7.

23. Valderrabano V, Perren T, Ryf C, et al. Snowboarder's talus fracture: treatment outcome of 20 cases after 3.5 years. Am J Sports Med 2005;33(6):871–80.

24. Snedden O, Christensen S, Krogsoe O. Fractures of the body of the talus. Acta Orthop Scand 1977;48:317–24.

25. Motto S. Stress fracture of the lateral process of the talus–a case report. Br J Sports Med 1993;27:275–6.

26. Sneppen O, Buhl O. Fracture of the talus: a study of its genesis and morphology based upon cases with associated ankle fractures. Acta Orthop Scand 1974;45: 307–20.

27. Chen YJ, Hsu RW, Shih HN, et al. Fracture of the entire posterior process of talus associated with subtalar dislocation: a case report. Foot Ankle Int 1996;17(4): 226–9.

28. Ebraheim NA, Padanilam TG, Wong FY. Posteromedial process fractures of the talus. Foot Ankle Int 1995;16(11):734–9.

29. Kanbe K, Kubota H, Hasegawa A, et al. Fracture of the posterior medial tubercle of the talus treated by internal fixation: a report of two cases. Foot Ankle Int 1995; 16(3):164–6.

30. Kim DH, Hrutkay JM, Samson MM. Fracture of the medial tubercle of the posterior process of the talus: a case report and literature review. Foot Ankle Int 1996; 17(3):186–8.

31. Nadim Y, Tosic A, Ebraheim NA. Open reduction and internal fixation of fracture of the posterior process of the talus: a case report and review of the literature. Foot Ankle Int 1999;20(1):50–2.

32. Nyska M, Howard CB, Matan Y, et al. Fracture of the posterior body of the talus– the hidden fracture. Arch Orthop Trauma Surg 1998;117(1–2):114–7.

33. Veazey BL, Heckman JD, Galindo MJ, et al. Excision of ununited fractures of the posterior process of the talus: a treatment for chronic posterior ankle pain. Foot Ankle Int 1992;13(8):453–7.

34. Wolf R, Heckman J. Case report: fracture of the posterior medial tubercle of the talus secondary to direct trauma. Foot Ankle Int 1998;19(4):255–8.

35. Kim D, Berkowitz M, Pressman D. Avulsion fractures of the medial tubercle of the posterior process. Foot Ankle Int 2003;24(2):172–5.

36. Giuffrida AY, Lin SS, Abidi N, et al. Pseudo os trigonum sign: missed posteromedial talar facet fracture. Foot Ankle Int 2003;24(8):642–9.

Management of Intra-Articular Fractures of the Calcaneus

Scott A. Swanson, MD[a], Michael P. Clare, MD[b], Roy W. Sanders, MD[c],*

KEYWORDS

• Calcaneus • Fracture • Intra-articular • Treatment

Since Malgaigne's first description in 1843,[1] fractures of the calcaneus have presented a significant challenge to orthopedic surgeons and patients alike. In describing the dismal results of early management of calcaneal fractures, Cotton and Wilson penned, "the man who breaks his heel bone is done."[2] Calcaneal fractures are the most common of tarsal bone fractures, and the majority are displaced intra-articular fractures, typically the result of falls from height or motor vehicle accidents. Calcaneal fractures affect primarily young men in their prime working years and result in a significant loss of economic productivity.[3–7] Although the development of modern imaging, surgical techniques, and fixation implants generally has improved functional outcome after these fractures, controversy continues to surround the management of these highly complex injuries. This article highlights current controversies and emphasizes treatment rationale and surgical approaches.

INTRA-ARTICULAR FRACTURES
Mechanism of Injury and Pathologic Anatomy

Displaced intra-articular fractures of the calcaneus generally occur as a result of high-energy trauma, with general agreement as to the pathomechanics involved.[4,8–11] With

One of the authors has received financial or material support (eg, equipment or services), commercially derived honoraria, or other nonresearch-related funding (eg, paid travel) from a commercial company or institution that relates directly or indirectly to the subject of this manuscript.

[a] Nebraska Orthopaedics and Sports Medicine, St. Elizabeth Medical Plaza, 575 South 70th Street Suite 200, Lincoln, NE 68510-2471, USA

[b] Florida Orthopaedic Institute, 13020 Telecom Parkway North, Tampa, FL 33637, USA

[c] Orthopaedic Trauma Service, Tampa General Hospital, The Florida Orthopaedic Institute, 4 Columbia Drive, Suite #710, Tampa, FL 33606, USA

* Corresponding author. Orthopaedic Trauma Service, Tampa General Hospital, The Florida Orthopaedic Institute, 4 Columbia Drive, Suite 710, Tampa, FL 33606.
E-mail address: ots1@aol.com (R. Sanders).

Foot Ankle Clin N Am 13 (2008) 659–678
doi:10.1016/j.fcl.2008.09.006
1083-7515/08/$ – see front matter © 2008 Elsevier Inc. All rights reserved.

a displaced intra-articular calcaneal fracture, the loss of height through the calcaneus results in a shortened and widened heel, typically with varus malalignment of the tuberosity. This loss of height is reflected in a decreased Böhler's angle, whereby the normal declination of the talus is diminished and the talus becomes relatively more horizontal, which may lead to a secondary loss of ankle dorsiflexion. As the superolateral fragment of the posterior facet is impacted plantarward, the thin lateral wall explodes laterally just posterior to the crucial angle of Gissane and may trap the peroneal tendons against the lateral malleolus; in some cases, a violent contracture of the peroneal tendons may avulse the tendon sheath from the fibula, resulting in an avulsion fracture of the lateral malleolus and dislocation of the peroneal tendons. The anterior process typically displaces superiorly, which limits subtalar joint motion directly by impinging against the lateral process of the talus.

Clarification of fragment terminology is necessary to understand the relevant pathoanatomy: the anterolateral fragment encompasses the lateral wall of the anterior process and may include a portion of the calcaneocuboid articular surface; the anterior main fragment is the large fragment anterior to the primary fracture line; the superomedial fragment (also known as the sustentacular or constant fragment) is found posterior to the primary fracture line and almost always remains attached to the talus through the deltoid ligament complex and, therefore, stable; the superolateral fragment is the lateral portion of the posterior facet, which is sheared from the remaining posterior facet in joint depression fractures; the tongue fragment refers to the superolateral fragment that remains attached to a portion of the posterior tuberosity in tongue-type fractures; and the posterior main fragment represents the posterior tuberosity (**Fig. 1**).

Diagnosis/Evaluation

The severity of fracture displacement and extent of soft tissue injury are related directly to the amount of energy absorbed by the limb in producing the injury. Higher-energy injuries, therefore, produce more severe soft tissue disruption and may result in an open fracture. Fracture bleeding into the tightly enveloped fascial planes surrounding the heel produces severe pain overlying the fracture and may result in a compartment syndrome of the foot. The normal skin creases typically disappear within several hours after the injury and in the event of extreme swelling, cleavage at the dermal-epidermal junction may produce fracture blisters. A high index of suspicion for associated injuries, including fractures of the lumbar spine, should be maintained.

Plain Radiography

Plain radiographic evaluation includes a lateral view of the hindfoot, an anteroposterior (A/P) view of the foot, an axial view of the heel,[12] and a mortise view of the ankle. The lateral view of the hindfoot reveals loss of height in the posterior facet, in which the articular surface is impacted within the body of the calcaneus and usually rotated anteriorly relative to the remaining subtalar joint; a decreased tuber angle of Böhler; and an increased crucial angle of Gissane seen in fracture patterns where the entire posterior facet is separated from the sustentaculum and depressed (**Fig. 2**). If only the lateral portion of the posterior facet is involved, the split in the articular surface is manifest as a double density,[13] in which case the tuber angle of Böhler and crucial angle of Gissane may remain normal (**Fig. 3**). The lateral view also allows delineation as to whether or not a fracture is a joint depression or tongue-type fracture.[4] The A/P view of the foot reveals anterolateral fragments and extension of fracture lines into the calcaneocuboid joint. The axial view of the heel shows loss of calcaneal length, increased width, and

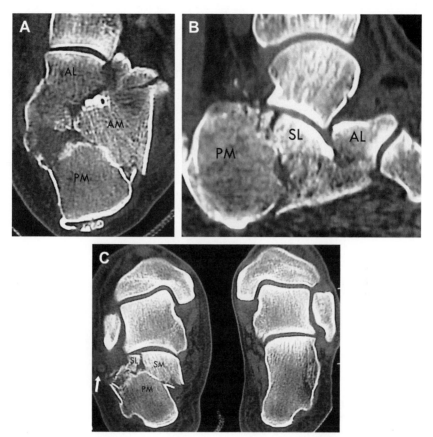

Fig. 1. Axial (*A*), sagittal (*B*), and semicoronal (*C*) CT images delineating typical calcaneal fracture fragments. AL, anterolateral; AM, anterior main; PM, posterior main; SL, superolateral; SM, superomedial.

(typically) varus angulation of the tuberosity fragment. A mortise view of the ankle usually demonstrates involvement of the posterior facet.

Computed Tomography

CT scanning is indicated if plain radiographs suggest intra-articular extension; images are obtained in 2- to 3-mm intervals in the axial, sagittal, and 30° semicoronal planes. The axial cuts show extension of fracture lines into the anterior process, calcaneocuboid joint, sustentaculum tali, and anteroinferior margin of the posterior facet. The sagittal reconstruction views demonstrate displacement of the tuberosity fragment; anterior process involvement, including superior displacement of the anterolateral fragment; anterior rotational displacement of the superolateral posterior facet fragment; and delineation of the fracture as a joint depression or tongue-type pattern.[4] The semicoronal images show displacement of articular fragments in the posterior facet, the sustentaculum tali, the extent of widening and shortening of the calcaneal body, expansion of the lateral calcaneal wall, and varus angulation of the tuberosity.

The images are assessed carefully in an attempt to provisionally understand the 3-D "personality" of the fracture. The fracture then is classified according to the Sanders classification to assist in determining the optimal method of treatment.[14]

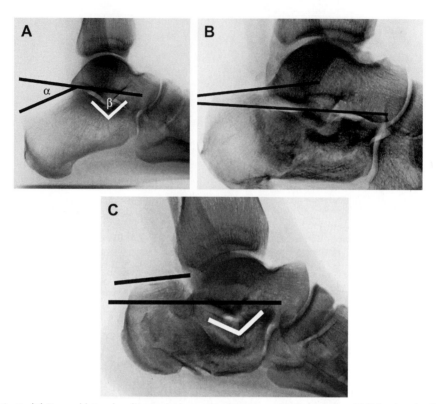

Fig. 2. (A) Normal lateral radiograph demonstrating normal tuber angle of Böhler (angle α) and crucial angle of Gissane (angle β). (B) Lateral injury radiograph showing decreased tuber angle of Böhler; note the marked loss of calcaneal height with relative horizontalization of talus. (C) Lateral injury radiograph with severe impaction of entire posterior facet; note decreased tuber angle of Böhler and increased crucial angle of Gissane.

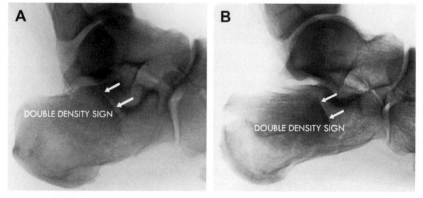

Fig. 3. Lateral injury radiographs with impaction of superolateral fragment manifest as double-density sign (*white arrows*) in (A) joint depression-type fracture pattern and (B) tongue-type fracture pattern.

TREATMENT
Nonoperative Treatment

Nonoperative management is best reserved for truly nondisplaced (Sanders type I) intra-articular fractures, as seen on CT scan, and fractures in patients who have severe peripheral vascular disease, type 1 diabetes mellitus, or other medical comorbidities prohibiting surgery and in elderly patients who are minimal (household) ambulators. Chronologic age is not necessarily a contraindication to surgical treatment, as many older patients are healthy and active well into their 70s.[15] Nonoperative treatment also may be necessary in certain instances because of injury severity, such as severe blistering, prolonged edema, or large open wounds, or in patients who have life-threatening injuries. In these instances, patients may be managed later for calcaneal malunion.[16]

Nonoperative treatment consists of initial splint immobilization, followed by conversion to an elastic compression stocking and prefabricated fracture boot locked in neutral flexion to allow early ankle and subtalar range-of-motion exercises. Weight bearing is not allowed for 10 to 12 weeks, until radiographic union is confirmed.

Operative Treatment

Operative treatment generally is indicated for displaced intra-articular fractures involving the posterior facet and ideally is performed within 3 weeks of injury before early fracture consolidation. Beyond this point, the fragments become increasingly difficult to separate to obtain an adequate reduction, and the articular cartilage may delaminate from the underlying subchondral bone. Surgery must be delayed, however, until the associated soft tissue swelling has dissipated adequately. Splint immobilization and limb elevation are performed initially and patients later are converted to a compression stocking and fracture boot. Full resolution of soft tissue edema is demonstrated by a positive wrinkle test,[17] indicating that surgical intervention may be undertaken safely.

Essex-Lopresti Technique for Tongue-type (Sanders Type IIC) Fractures

Patients are placed in the lateral decubitus position and, under fluoroscopic guidance in the lateral view, two terminally threaded guide pins are inserted in the posterosuperior edge of the posterior tuberosity and advanced toward the anterior-inferior edge of the displaced posterior facet.[18] With the dorsum of the foot held in the palm of one hand and the guide pins with the palm of the other hand, the Essex-Lopresti maneuver is performed in three steps. First, the foot is forced into varus to unlock the primary fracture. Second, the guide pins are levered plantarward while simultaneously plantarflexing the midfoot. Finally, the foot is forced into valgus to bring the posterior facet adjacent to the sustentaculum. The reduction of the tongue fragment is confirmed fluoroscopically with the midfoot still held in plantarflexion, and the guide pins are advanced into the anterior process region. A Brodén's view[19] is obtained, assessing the reduction of the articular surface, and guide pin position is confirmed on the lateral, axial, and A/P views. Definitive fixation is achieved with two large cannulated screws or multiple small fragment lag screws (**Fig. 4**).

If the tongue fragment fails to disimpact, a small periosteal elevator may be used through a small stab incision to disimpact the fragment and assist with reduction. If widening remains between the sustentaculum and the articular portion of the tongue fragment in the coronal plane, a small fragment lag screw may be placed in the sustentaculum to narrow the posterior facet (**Fig. 4**). In the event of an irreducible tongue

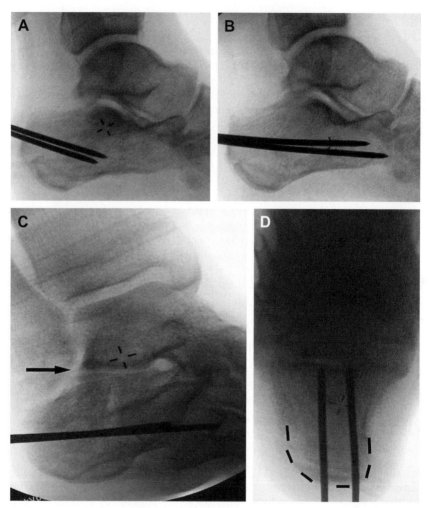

Fig. 4. Tongue-type calcaneal fracture treated with Essex-Lopresti reduction maneuver. (*A*) Initial placement of guide pins. (*B–D*) Alignment after reduction and advancement of guide pins. (*E–G*) Definitive stabilization of tongue-type calcaneal fracture with multiple small fragment screws.

fragment, the reduction is converted to a formal open reduction and a standard extensile lateral approach is used.

The percutaneous incisions are closed and supportive splint is placed. Patients are later converted to a compression stocking and fracture boot to allow early ankle and subtalar range-of-motion exercises; weight bearing is not permitted until 10 to 12 weeks postoperatively.

Extensile Lateral Approach for Joint Depression Fractures

Patients are placed in the lateral decubitus position on a beanbag. Attention to detail with respect to placement of the incision and gentle soft tissue handling is of paramount importance, as soft tissue complications remain a major source of morbidity with these injuries.[20,21] A full-thickness, subperiosteal flap is raised and 1.6-mm

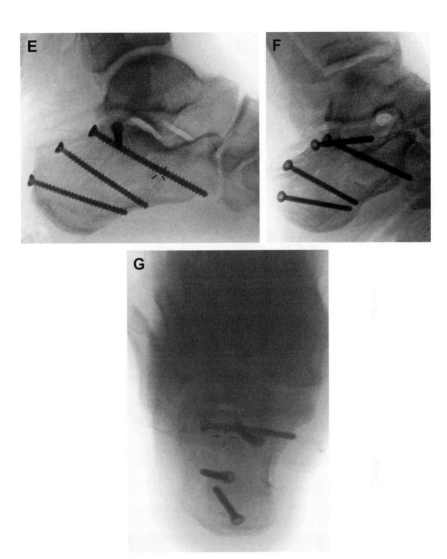

Fig. 4. (*continued*)

Kirschner wires (K-wires) are placed in the fibula, talar neck, and cuboid, for retraction of the subperiosteal flap.

The expanded lateral wall fragment and impacted superolateral articular fragment are mobilized carefully and preserved in saline on the back table, which affords exposure of the superomedial fragment and the obliquely oriented primary fracture line (**Fig. 5**). A blunt periosteal elevator is introduced into the primary fracture line and levered plantarward, thereby disimpacting the posterior main fragment from the superomedial fragment and restoring calcaneal height and length along the medial calcaneal wall.[22] A 4.5-mm Schantz pin is placed in the posterior-inferior corner of the calcaneal tuberosity for further manipulation.[23]

The anterior process fragments are next pulled inferiorly and provisionally secured with 1.6-mm K-wires. There often is variability in fracture lines through the anterior process in that there may be three separate fragments and, as the anterolateral fragment

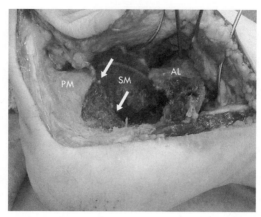

Fig. 5. Intraoperative view after excision of lateral wall fragment and superolateral fragment. Mobilization through primary fracture line (*white arrows*). AL, anterolateral; SM, superomedial; PM, posterior main.

is reduced, the central fragment may remain displaced superiorly. In this instance, a lamina spreader may be used to facilitate reduction of the central fragment. A transverse fracture line may be present through the crucial angle of Gissane, in essence rotating the superomedial fragment beneath the anterior main fragment. In this case, before reduction of the superolateral articular fragment, the superomedial fragment must be derotated, reduced, and provisionally stabilized to the anterior main fragment to prevent malrotation of the entire posterior facet articular surface.

The superolateral fragment (Sanders type II fracture) is brought back into the wound and two parallel 1.6-mm K-wires are placed like toothpicks to facilitate reduction; in the event of two separate fragments (Sanders type III fracture), the central articular fragment is first reduced to the superomedial fragment and stabilized with 1.5-mm bioresorbable poly-lactic acid pins. The protruding ends of the bioresorbable pins are removed flush with the bony surface with a handheld electrocautery unit. The superolateral (lateral-most articular) fragment then is reduced and provisionally stabilized with 1.6-mm k-wires to the central and superomedial fragments. The articular fragments must be reduced precisely such that (superior-inferior) height, (anterior-posterior) rotation, and coronal plane (varus-valgus) alignment are correct. The articular reduction is verified through "window" visualization: the superolateral and superomedial fragments should align anteriorly and posteriorly. Failure to visualize the posterior facet from both sides of the window may lead to malreduction of the fragments in the sagittal plane (**Fig. 6**).

At this point, the posterior edge of the anterolateral fragment should key into the anterior-inferior edge of the superolateral fragment, indicating restoration of the crucial angle of Gissane; the lateral wall and the body of the calcaneus should align with simple valgus manipulation of the Schantz pin; and the previously excised lateral wall fragment should anatomically reduce, confirming at the least that the lateral column is anatomically restored. The reduction then is confirmed by intraoperative fluoroscopy, including lateral, Brodén's, and axial views (**Fig. 7**).

The posterior facet is secured with 3.5-mm cortical lag screws placed just beneath the articular surface angling toward the sustentaculum. A low-profile lateral neutralization plate is then selected and secured with 4.0-mm cancellous screws, starting with the distal-most screw holes overlying the anterior process. The oblique orientation of

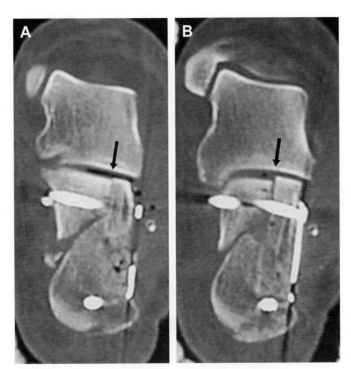

Fig. 6. Sagittal plane rotational malalignment of superolateral fragment from inadequate window visualization. (*A*) Postoperative semicoronal CT image through anterior portion of posterior facet: intra-articular alignment appears near anatomic (*arrow*). (*B*) Postoperative semicoronal CT image through posterior portion of posterior facet: note intra-articular step-off (*arrow*).

the calcaneocuboid articulation is accommodated by aiming slightly posteriorly. Screw placement on power brings the plate to bone, thus restoring calcaneal width. Next, the calcaneal tuberosity is secured to the plate while maintaining a simultaneous lateral-to-medial force on the plate, and a valgus-directed force on the tuberosity (**Fig. 8**). The main components of the calcaneus (anterior process, posterior tuberosity, and articular surface) are further secured to the plate such that a minimum of two screws traverses each component (**Fig. 9**).

The peroneal tendons are assessed for stability by advancing a Freer elevator within the peroneal tendon sheath to the level of the lateral malleolus and levering anteriorly. If the superior peroneal retinaculum and tendon sheath are unstable, the elevator easily slides anterior to the fibula, in which case a tendon sheath repair is required (**Fig. 10**). The full-thickness flap is closed over a deep drain with deep #0 absorbable sutures placed starting at the proximal and distal ends and progressing toward the apex of the incision. They are hand-tied sequentially in similar fashion so as to eliminate tension at the apex of the incision. The skin layer is closed with 3-0 monofilament suture using the modified Allgöwer-Donati technique.

After splint immobilization, patients are converted back into a compression stocking and fracture boot at 3 weeks postoperatively, and early ankle and subtalar range-of-motion exercises are begun. The sutures are removed once the incision is fully sealed and dry, typically at 3 to 4 weeks; however, weight bearing is not initiated until 10 to 12 weeks postoperatively.

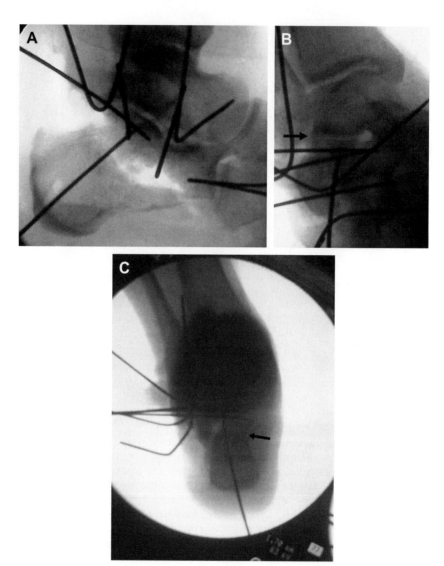

Fig. 7. Intraoperative (*A*) lateral, (*B*) Brodén's, and (*C*) axial fluoroscopic images demonstrating provisional reduction; note anatomic alignment of posterior facet articular surface (*B*) and restoration of calcaneal height and length (*C*) (*black arrows*).

Combined (Open/Closed) Techniques for Split Tongue Fractures

Intra-articular tongue-type patterns (Sanders types IIA or B and III) require an extensile lateral approach due to the pull of the Achilles tendon on the fragment, which often precludes reduction of the lateral articular tongue fragment in proper sagittal plane rotation. In this instance, the Essex-Lopresti reduction technique is performed on the tongue fragment in an open fashion with a 4.5-mm Schantz pin placed percutaneously into the tongue fragment, which neutralizes the deforming forces of the Achilles tendon and allows anatomic reduction of the articular surface in the sagittal plane (**Fig. 11**). The remainder of the procedure is then completed (as described previously).

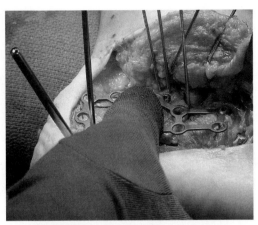

Fig. 8. Fixation of calcaneal tuberosity: simultaneous lateral-to-medial force on plate (applied by surgeon's thumb) and valgus-directed force on undersurface of tuberosity (applied by surgeon's long and ring fingers).

Minimally Invasive Techniques

Concerns over wound complications have prompted some to develop minimally invasive approaches to treating intra-articular calcaneus fractures. The indications for a minimally invasive approach include the emergent reduction and stabilization of fractures with severe or impending soft tissue compromise from displaced fracture fragments. Closed or percutaneous reduction and external fixation supplemented by K-wire fixation may be followed by standard open treatment if the soft tissues are amenable within 2 to 3 weeks. For those patients who have relative contraindications to open surgery, such as heavy smokers or patients who have severe peripheral vascular disease or poorly controlled diabetes, minimally invasive approaches may be used as definitive treatment. In general, small incisions are used for placement of Schantz pins and small periosteal elevators in assisting with the reduction, followed by multiple small fragment screws axially and laterally (**Fig. 12**). Tongue-type fractures are particularly amenable to these approaches, with investigators reporting good results with minimally invasive reduction techniques combined with small fragment fixation for tongue-type fractures fractures.[18,24]

With experience, these applications have been expanded to include treatment of joint depression fractures.[25] Forgon[26] described a method of 3-point skeletal traction applied to the tuberosity, talus, and cuboid, using ligamentotaxis to manipulate the main fragments. The depressed posterior facet is elevated percutaneously with a K-wire introduced laterally. The reduction is confirmed on fluoroscopy and the fragments are fixed with percutaneously placed lag screws. Some have described percutaneous or mini–open reduction with use of small wire circular external fixators.[27,28] The use of temporary uniplanar, unilateral external fixation also is described.[29] The early results of these minimally invasive approaches are comparable to traditional open methods.

A major concern surrounding the application of minimally invasive approaches is the potential for incomplete or malreduction of the posterior facet. Rammelt and colleagues[25] have used subtalar arthroscopy successfully to assist in judging the quality of articular reduction. As discussed later, intraoperative CT scanning may improve the execution of minimally invasive techniques. Minimally invasive techniques should be

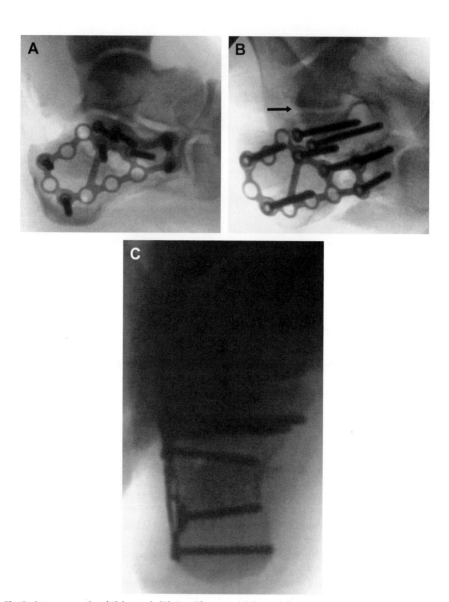

Fig. 9. Intraoperative (*A*) lateral, (*B*) Brodén's, and (*C*) axial fluoroscopic images demonstrating definitive fixation and final reduction.

reserved for simple fracture patterns. Before attempting these technically demanding approaches, surgeons should be thoroughly familiar with the pathoanatomy of intra-articular calcaneal fractures and have mastery of traditional open techniques.

Fracture/Dislocation Patterns

Fracture-dislocation patterns are rare,[30–32] and occur when the superolateral fragment remains contiguous with the lateral wall and posterior tuberosity. The resulting large lateral fragment dislocates laterally and is forcefully driven into the talofibular joint, often producing a fracture of the lateral malleolus. Because of the generally high-energy

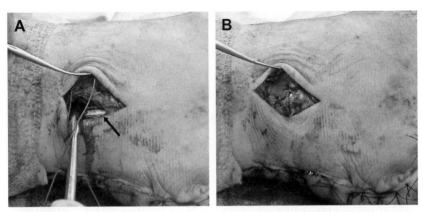

Fig. 10. Superior peroneal retinaculum repair of dislocated peroneal tendons after calcaneal stabilization. (*A*) Suture anchors placed in distal fibula with sutures passed through false pouch anteriorly and tied with peroneal tendons held reduced in peroneal groove (*black arrow*). (*B*) Final construct with stable tendons.

nature of the injury, the peroneal tendons typically dislocate anteriorly, and the lateral ligamentous complex of the ankle joint is disrupted. With recoil of the limb, there is inversion of the hindfoot through the ankle joint, which is manifest radiographically as increased lateral talar tilt. CT evaluation reveals the typical fracture-dislocation pattern.

The fracture pattern is most commonly a simple two-part split fracture, such that as the dislocation is reduced, the articular fragments typically align anatomically. As with most dislocations, the sooner it is reduced, the easier the reduction tends to be; with delayed treatment, a formal open reduction usually is required. With patients in the lateral decubitus position, a blunt periosteal elevator is introduced through a small stab incision at the superior edge of the lateral tuberosity fragment, and advanced inferiorly along the medial surface of the fragment until positioned at the inferolateral edge of the

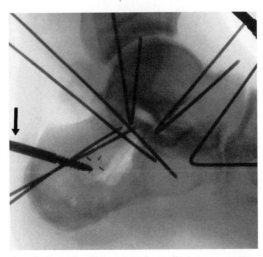

Fig. 11. Essex-Lopresti technique for intra-articular split tongue pattern; note Schantz pin within tongue fragment (*arrow*) to neutralize pull of Achilles tendon.

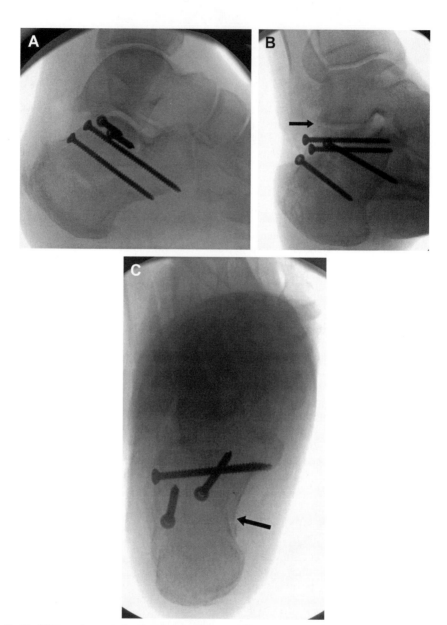

Fig. 12. (A) Percutaneous fixation for Sanders type IIB tongue-type fracture. The patient also sustained a contralateral proximal humerus fracture and a spinal cord contusion and developed a pulmonary embolus requiring anticoagulation, necessitating percutaneous reduction and fixation. Note (B) anatomic reduction of posterior facet (*black arrow*) but (C) residual shortening and varus malalignment of tuberosity (*black arrow*).

talus within the subtalar joint. The lateral tuberosity fragment is then gently levered plantarward—the fragment typically reduces once it clears the inferolateral edge of the talus. Definitive fixation of the fracture typically may be completed in percutaneous fashion with cortical lag screws, in combination with repair of the lateral ligamentous complex of the ankle and superior peroneal retinaculum. The limb is immobilized for 6 weeks postoperatively for healing of the soft tissue repair; weight bearing is initiated at 10 to 12 weeks.

Open Calcaneus Fractures

Open fractures of the calcaneus are distinct injuries relative to closed fractures, and generally are associated with a higher complication rate, including deep infection, osteomyelitis, and need for amputation.[33–36] The degree of soft tissue injury is the most important variable predicting outcome, and the incidence of major complications seems to increase with increasing severity of the soft-tissue injury. Open fractures of the calcaneus may present with a puncture wound medially from a spike of bone or present with a more significant soft tissue injury, typically laterally or posteriorly.

Treatment includes antibiotic prophylaxis, and irrigation and débridement of the wound. All open type I and those type II fractures with a medial wound are treated with delayed open reduction and internal fixation once the soft tissues are suitable for surgery. Open type II fractures with a nonmedial wound and all open type IIIA wounds are treated with percutaneous stabilization or external fixation; all open type IIIB wounds are best managed by late reconstruction.[35]

Open Reduction with Internal Fixation/Primary Arthrodesis for Sanders Type IV Fractures

Open reduction with internal fixation (ORIF) with primary subtalar arthrodesis is indicated only for highly comminuted intra-articular fractures, in which the articular surface is determined to be nonreconstructable.[14,37] Standard ORIF techniques are used, such that calcaneal height, length, and overall morphology are fully reestablished. The remaining articular cartilage is removed from the corresponding surfaces of the posterior facet and the subchondral surfaces are drilled with a 2.5-mm drill bit for vascular ingrowth, and supplemental cancellous allograft is placed within the subtalar joint. With the subtalar joint held in neutral alignment, definitive fixation for the arthrodesis is obtained with two large (6.5–8.0 mm) cannulated screws placed from posterior to anterior in diverging fashion perpendicular to the plane of the posterior facet (**Fig. 13**). One of the 3.5-mm cortical lag screws may need to be removed and subsequently redirected to allow placement of the larger cannulated screws; ideally,

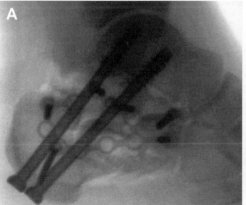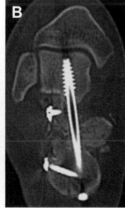

Fig. 13. (*A*) Intraoperative lateral and (*B*) postoperative semicoronal CT images demonstrating ORIF and primary subtalar arthrodesis; note restoration of calcaneal height and overall morphology.

however, the lag screw placed through the plate is preserved so as to maintain continuity between the posterior facet and the remainder of the calcaneus. Patients are maintained in serial short-leg casts for 10 to 12 weeks, at which point radiographic union of the fracture and the arthrodesis is confirmed.

Intraoperative 3-D Fluoroscopy

Standard fluoroscopy has limitations in terms of precise definition of articular reduction and implant position. For this reason, many surgeons obtain a postoperative CT scan. In the event of articular incongruity or implant malposition, surgeons are forced to accept the result or return to the operating room. To address these concerns, some centers are investigating the use of a mobile isocentric C-arm with 3-D imaging. Several studies have shown that intraoperative 3-D fluoroscopy has greater sensitivity and specificity than standard fluoroscopy for identifying articular incongruity and implant malposition with only minimal additional operating room time.[38–40] 3-D fluoroscopy has been shown to be equivalent to CT.[40] Intraoperative 3-D fluoroscopy may obviate postoperative CT scans and may improve outcomes in the treatment of intra-articular calcaneus fractures. Its use as an adjuvant to minimally invasive approaches is particularly appealing. 3-D fluoroscopy is not yet widely available, and further study is needed to define which fractures and surgical approaches are best served by its use.

Locking Plates

The introduction of locking plate technology has been an important advance in the treatment of complex, periarticular fractures and fractures in osteopenic bone. Recently, several calcaneal locking plates have been introduced. In cadaveric models, locked plates generally have increased the stability of fracture fixation,[41] with polyaxially locked screws performing best.[42] One study showed no biomechanical advantage with locking plate fixation in a cadaver model of type IIB fractures.[43] To date, no studies have demonstrated clinical superiority of locked calcaneal plates to non-locked, low-profile neutralization plates. The indications for locking plates in the treatment of calcaneus fractures are still being defined but may include use in highly comminuted fractures, the elderly, or those who have particularly poor bone stock (**Fig. 14**).

COMPLICATIONS
Delayed Wound Healing/Wound Dehiscence

The most common complication after surgical treatment of a calcaneal fracture is wound dehiscence, which occurs in up to 25% of cases.[14,23,34,36,44–47] Despite easy approximation at the time of surgical closure, the wound may later separate, typically at the apex of the incision, even up to 4 weeks after surgery. The majority of wounds ultimately heal, as deep infection and osteomyelitis develop in 1% to 4% of closed fractures.[14,34,44–46,48]

If a wound dehiscence should occur, all range-of-motion exercises are discontinued to prevent further wound separation. The wound is managed with serial whirlpool treatments, damp-to-dry dressing changes, and oral antibiotics. Alternatively, cast immobilization may be instituted with window access for dressing changes. Once the wound seals, range-of-motion exercises are reinstituted. A negative pressure device (Vacuum Assisted Closure, KCI, San Antonio, Texas) may be used for recalcitrant wounds.[48]

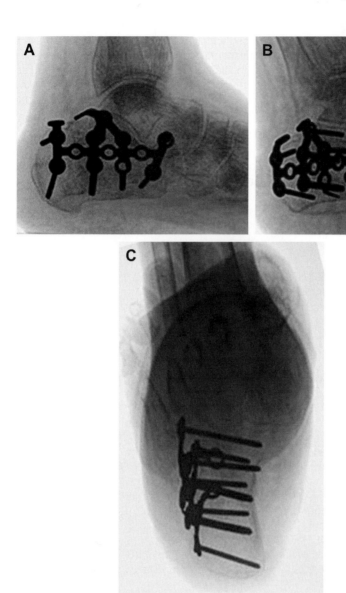

Fig. 14. (*A–C*) Locking plate fixation in patient who had a history of seizure disorder and osteopenic bone.

Posttraumatic Arthritis

A principal goal of internal fixation is anatomic restoration of the posterior facet articular surface. Posttraumatic arthritis still may develop, however, even in cases of a truly anatomic reduction, as a result of cartilage damage at the time of injury.[17] In this instance, because calcaneal height and morphology already have been restored, implant removal and an in situ subtalar arthrodesis may be performed.[17,49–51] Radnay and colleagues[51] performed a retrospective cohort study comparing outcomes for patients initially treated by open reduction and internal fixation who required late subtalar arthrodesis with patients treated nonoperatively who went onto develop calcaneal malunions. The latter group was treated according to the protocol of Stephens and Sanders with reconstruction and subtalar arthrodesis.[52] The investigators reported superior results in those patients who had initial surgical treatment, suggesting that restoration of calcaneal height, length, and morphology is beneficial to outcome even in the event of late posttraumatic arthritis, at which point an in situ arthrodesis is performed.

SUMMARY

The treatment of calcaneal fractures has evolved over time. Despite understanding the pathomechanics involved, these fractures remain difficult to treat. Advances in imaging and surgical technology have enabled experienced fracture surgeons to obtain consistent results. Obtaining anatomic reduction at the time of surgery is of paramount importance. Minimally invasive approaches and the emergence of new technology may aid surgeons who treat these complex fractures.

REFERENCES

1. Malgaigne J-F. Operative surgery, based on normal and pathological anatomy. Frederick Brittan (trans). 1st edition. Philadelphia: Blanchard and Lea; 1851.
2. Cotton FJ, Wilson LT. Fractures of the Os Calcis. Boston Med Surg J 1908;159: 559–65.
3. Aaron AD. Ankle fusion: a retrospective review. Orthopedics 1990;13:1249–54.
4. Essex-Lopresti P. The mechanism, reduction technique, and results in fractures of the os calcis. Br J Surg 1952;39:395–419.
5. Lindsay WRN, Dewar FP. Fractures of the os calcis. Am J Surg 1958;95:555–76.
6. Parkes JC II. The nonreductive treatment for fractures of the os calcis. Orthop Clin North Am 1973;4:193–5.
7. Widen A. Fractures of the calcaneus: a clinical study with special reference to the technique and results of open reduction. Acta Chir Scand Suppl 1954;188:1–119.
8. Burdeaux BD. Reduction of calcaneal fractures by the McReynolds medial approach technique and its experimental basis. Clin Orthop Relat Res 1983; 177:87–103.
9. Carr JB, Hamilton JJ, Bear LS. Experimental intraarticular calcaneal fractures: anatomic basis for a new classification. Foot Ankle 1989;10:81–7.
10. Palmer I. The mechanism and treatment of fractures of the calcaneus. J Bone Joint Surg Am 1948;30:2–8.
11. Thoren O. Os calcis fractures. Acta Orthop Scand 11(Suppl) 1964;70:1–116.
12. Isherwood I. A radiographic approach to the subtalar joint. J Bone Joint Surg Br 1961;43:566–74.
13. Sanders R. Displaced intra-articular fractures of the calcaneus. J Bone Joint Surg Am 2000;82:225–50.
14. Sanders R, Fortin P, DiPasquale T, et al. Operative treatment in 120 displaced intraarticular calcaneal fractures. Results using a prognostic computed tomography scan classification. Clin Orthop Relat Res 1993;290:87–95.
15. Herscovici D Jr, Widmaier J, Scaduto JM, et al. Operative treatment of calcaneal fractures in elderly patients. J Bone Joint Surg Am 2005;87:1260–4.
16. Clare MP, Lee WE III, Sanders RW. Intermediate to long-term results of a treatment protocol for calcaneal fracture malunions. J Bone Joint Surg Am 2005;87:963–73.
17. Sanders R. Intra-articular fractures of the calcaneus: present state of the art. J Orthop Trauma 1992;6:252–65.
18. Tornetta P III. The Essex-Lopresti reduction for calcaneal fractures revisited. J Orthop Trauma 1998;12:469–73.

19. Broden B. Roentgen examination of the subtaloid joint in fractures of the calcaneus. Acta Radiol 1949;31:85–91.
20. Borrelli J Jr, Lashgari C. Vascularity of the lateral calcaneal flap: a cadaveric injection study. J Orthop Trauma 1999;13:73–7.
21. Gould N. Lateral approach to the os calcis. Foot Ankle 1984;4:218–20.
22. Eastwood DM, Langkamer VG, Atkins RM. Intra-articular fractures of the calcaneum. Part II: open reduction and internal fixation by the extended lateral transcalcaneal approach. J Bone Joint Surg Br 1993;75:189–95.
23. Benirschke SK, Sangeorzan BJ. Extensive intraarticular fractures of the foot. Surgical management of calcaneal fractures. Clin Orthop 1993;291:128–34.
24. Sangeorzan BJ, Ringler JR. Minimally invasive reduction and small fragment fixation of tongue-type calcaneus fractures, OTA 17th Annual Meeting, poster # 46. Orthopaedic Trauma Association 2001:17, poster # 46,275.
25. Rammelt S, Amlang M, Barthel S, et al. Minimally-invasive treatment of calcaneal fractures. Injury 2004;35(Suppl 2):SB55–63.
26. Forgon M. Closed reduction and percutaneous osteosynthesis: technique and results in 265 calcaneal fractures. In: Tscherne H, Schatzker J, editors. Major fractures of the pilon, the talus, and the calcaneus. Berlin: Springer Verlag; 1992.
27. McGarvey WC, Burris MW, Clanton TO, et al. Calcaneal fractures: indirect reduction and external fixation. Foot Ankle Int 2006;27(7):494–9.
28. Emara KM, Allam MF. Management of calcaneal fracture using the Ilizarov technique. Clin Orthop Relat Res 2005;439:215–20.
29. Magnan B, Bortolazzi R, Marangon A, et al. External fixation for displaced intraarticular fractures of the calcaneum. J Bone Joint Surg Br 2006;88(11):1474–9.
30. Eastwood DM, Maxwell AC, Atkins RM. Fracture of the lateral malleolus with talar tilt: primarily a calcaneal fracture not an ankle injury. Injury 1993;24:109–12.
31. Ebraheim NA, Elgafy H, Sabry FF, et al. Calcaneus fractures with subluxation of the posterior facet. A surgical indication. Clin Orthop 2000;377:210–6.
32. Turner NS, Haidukewych GJ. Locked fracture dislocation of the calcaneus treated with minimal open reduction and percutaneous fixation: a report of two cases and review of the literature. Foot Ankle Int 2003;24:796–800.
33. Aldridge JM III, Easley M, Nunley JA. Open calcaneal fractures: results of operative treatment. J Orthop Trauma 2004;18:7–11.
34. Benirschke SK, Kramer PA. Wound healing complications in closed and open calcaneal fractures. J Orthop Trauma 2004;18:1–6.
35. Heier KA, Infante AF, Walling AK, et al. Open fractures of the calcaneus: soft-tissue injury determines outcome. J Bone Joint Surg Am 2003;85:2276–82.
36. Folk JW, Starr AJ, Early JS. Early wound complications of operative treatment of calcaneus fractures: analysis of 190 fractures. J Orthop Trauma 1999;13:369–72.
37. Clare MP, Sanders RW. Open reduction and internal fixation with primary subtalar arthrodesis for Sanders type IV calcaneus fractures. Tech Foot Ankle Surg 2004; 3:250–7.
38. Richter M, Geerling J, Zech S, et al. Intraoperative three-dimensional imaging with a motorized mobile C-arm (SIREMOBIL ISO-C-3D) in foot and ankle trauma care: a preliminary report. J Orthop Trauma 2005;19(4):259–66.
39. Atesok K, Finkelstein J, Khoury A, et al. The use of intraoperative three-dimensional imaging (ISO-C-3D) in fixation of intraarticular fractures. Injury 2007;38(10):1163–9 [Epub 2007 Sep 19].
40. Kendoff D, Citak M, Gardner M, et al. Three-dimensional fluoroscopy for evaluation of articular reduction and screw placement in calcaneal fractures. Foot Ankle Int 2007;28(11):1165–71.

41. Stoffel K, Booth G, Rohrl SM, et al. A comparison of conventional versus locking plates in intraarticular calcaneus fractures: a biomechanical study in human cadavers. Clin Biomech (Bristol, Avon) 2007;22(1):100–5 [Epub 2006 Sep 27].

42. Richter M, Droste P, Goesling T, et al. Polyaxially-locked plate screws increase stability of fracture fixation in an experimental model of calcaneal fracture. J Bone Joint Surg Br 2006;88(9):1257–63.

43. Redfern DJ, Oliveira ML, Campbell JT, et al. A biomechanical comparison of locking and nonlocking plates for the fixation of calcaneal fractures. Foot Ankle Int 2006;27(3):196–201.

44. Harvey EJ, Grujic L, Early JS, et al. Morbidity associated with ORIF of intra-articular calcaneus fractures using a lateral approach. Foot Ankle Int 2001;22:868–73.

45. Howard JL, Buckley R, McCormack R, et al. Complications following management of displaced intra-articular calcaneal fractures: a prospective randomized trial comparing open reduction internal fixation with nonoperative management. J Orthop Trauma 2003;17:241–9.

46. Levin LS, Nunley JA. The management of soft-tissue problems associated with calcaneal fractures. Clin Orthop 1993;290:151–60.

47. Lim EV, Leung JP. Complications of intraarticular calcaneal fractures. Clin Orthop 2001;391:7–16.

48. Herscovici D Jr, Sanders RW, Scatudo JM, et al. Vacuum-assisted wound closure (VAC therapy) for the management of patients with high-energy soft tissue injuries. J Orthop Trauma 2003;17:683–8.

49. Flemister AS Jr, Infante AF, Sanders RW, et al. Subtalar arthrodesis for complications of intra-articular calcaneal fractures. Foot Ankle Int 2000;21:392–9.

50. Sanders R, Fortin P, Walling A. Subtalar arthrodesis following calcaneal fracture. Orthop Trans 1991;15:656.

51. Radnay CS, Clare MP, Sanders RW, et al. Subtalar fusion after displaced intra-articular calcaneal fractures: Does initial operative treatment matter? J Bone Joint Surg Am 2009;91(3); in press.

52. Stephens HM, Sanders R. Calcaneal malunions: results of a prognostic computed tomography classification system. Foot Ankle Int 1996;17:395–401.

Chopart Fractures and Dislocations

Michael P. Swords, DO[a],*, Matthew Schramski, DO[b],
Kyle Switzer, DO[b], Scott Nemec, DO[b]

KEYWORDS

- Chopart • Midfoot • Talus • Navicular
- Cuboid • Fracture

The Chopart joint is named after Francois Chopart (1743–1795), who described the use of the talonavicular and calcaneocuboid articulations as a practical level for amputation.[1] Injuries to the midfoot and Chopart complex most commonly occur as a result of high-energy trauma. Motor vehicle accidents (MVAs) and crushing injuries produce most of these injuries. Cadaveric studies have demonstrated that in motor vehicle collisions forces can be greater in Chopart's joints than in the ankle.[2] Axial loading also can result in significant midfoot trauma. Examination of all patients suspected of having midfoot injuries should be thorough. Particular diligence is necessary in the trauma population, because foot injuries can be missed, and injuries to the midfoot and Chopart's joints occur in nearly 10% of polytrauma patients who suffer foot or ankle injuries in MVAs.[3] Gross deformities often accompany dislocations and severe crushing injuries. Soft tissue injuries are fairly common because of the thin soft tissue envelope. Ankle and lower extremity injuries can occur in conjunction with midfoot injuries, and care should be taken to identify them if present. All dislocations should be reduced emergently if possible. Open wounds should be covered with saline-soaked gauze, and the extremity should be splinted. Radiographic assessment is essential and should include imaging of both the foot and ankle as a preliminary screen. In more comminuted injuries to Chopart joints, the bony architecture can be altered to the extent that reduction is not possible because of the lack of bony stability. In these situations, external fixation can be used to maintain more normal alignment of the foot while waiting for the soft tissues to allow open fixation techniques, typically for 1 to 2 weeks. CT can be invaluable in understanding the extent of injury and planning operative fixation. Often, fractures not readily apparent on conventional radiographs are identified on CT scanning.

[a] Section of Orthopedics, Sparrow Health System, Mid Michigan Orthopedic Institute, Michigan State University College of Osteopathic Medicine, 830 W. Lake Lansing Suite 190, East Lansing, MI 48823, USA
[b] Department of Medical Education, Ingham Regional Medical Center, Michigan State University College of Osteopathic Medicine, 401 W. Greenlawn Avenue, Lansing, MI 48901, USA
* Corresponding author.
E-mail address: foot.trauma@gmail.com (M.P. Swords).

Foot Ankle Clin N Am 13 (2008) 679–693
doi:10.1016/j.fcl.2008.08.004
1083-7515/08/$ – see front matter © 2008 Elsevier Inc. All rights reserved.

foot.theclinics.com

ANATOMY AND FUNCTION OF THE MIDFOOT

The midfoot provides a crucial link locking the hindfoot to the forefoot as is necessary in normal gait. When the hindfoot is everted, the two Chopart joints are parallel, allowing flexibility; when the hindfoot is inverted, the joints come out of their parallel configuration, stiffening the joints for push off.[4] Talonavicular motion is closely linked to subtalar motion and motion through the calcaneocuboid joint, allowing the foot to invert and evert during gait.[5] The head of the talus rotates in its articulation with the navicular surface in a mobile fashion. For these reasons the talonavicular joint, along with the ankle and subtalar joints, is considered an essential joint for normal foot biomechanics and function.[6] The navicular joint also articulates with the three cuneiform joints, and on occasion a fourth articular facet is present between the navicular and the cuboid. The naviculocuneiform articulations are quite limited in motion, providing stability for the transverse tarsal arch and the longitudinal medial column. Loss of this support leads to collapse of the normal arches of the foot. The cuboid articulates in a mobile fashion with the anterior process of the calcaneus. Distally, articulations between the cuboid and the fourth and fifth metatarsal bases are extremely mobile and help the foot accommodate to varied walking surfaces. Salvage procedures for late reconstruction of the cuboid metatarsal articulation are unpredictable and generally are poorly tolerated. The cuboid and navicular are key structures in maintaining appropriate lengths of the medial and lateral columns. It is important to restore normal anatomy, even in highly comminuted injuries, because of the high potential for disability, pain, and loss of function that can occur if neglected.

Medial Column Injuries

Talar head injuries

The talar head projects anteromedially from the talar neck to its articulation with the navicular. Most of the talar head is covered by articular cartilage. The navicular articulation rotates around the talar head, comprising the acetabulum pedis. Blood supply to the talar head is provided proximally through intraosseus branches from the artery of the tarsal sinus and by branches from the dorsalis pedis and travels distally to the talar head. Fractures can deprive the articular fragments of necessary blood supply, resulting in avascular necrosis (**Fig. 1**).

Fractures to the talar head arise from axial loads applied through the navicular bone to the head of the talus. There are often substantial compressive forces resulting in comminution of the talar head and navicular articular surfaces. Significant impaction of the talar head can occur from the axial load as the talar head collides with the navicular articular surface or as the head dislocates, as typically seen in talonavicular fracture dislocations (**Fig. 2**). All displaced talar head fractures require open reduction and fixation to restore bony contact and articular congruity. Dislocations also can result in significant shear injuries to the talar head, essentially peeling the articular cartilage off the talar head. Injuries with significant impaction and articular cartilage loss that are not reconstructable are best treated with primary arthrodesis.

More severe injuries generally are associated with talonavicular dislocations, which can result in significant shortening of the medial column. During operative fixation it often is necessary to use an external fixator or other form of distractor to create the space necessary to visualize and reconstruct the talar head (**Fig. 3**). Partial articular injuries can be reconstructed after adequate distraction. Fixation typically consists of small or mini fragment screws inserted through the articular surface. The screw heads are countersunk to avoid further injury to the articular surface with motion. If the fracture extends more proximally, plate fixation is an option. Mini blade plates

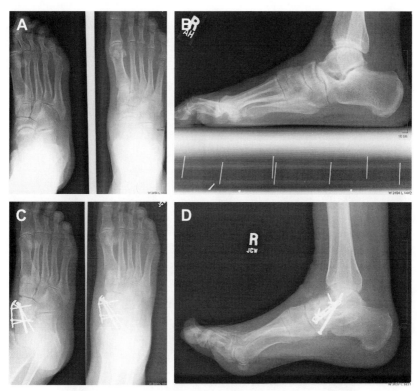

Fig. 1. (*A*) Anteroposterior (AP), oblique, and (*B*) lateral radiographs of a 60-year-old man. The patient developed avascular necrosis because of the disruption of the blood supply to the articular fragment. (*C, D*) The patient was treated with resection of avascular bone, iliac crest bone grafting, and arthrodesis.

and traditional plating techniques are available, as are newer locking constructs. After fixation, the subtalar joint and talonavicular stability should be assessed. If instability exists, an external fixator may be applied to maintain stability, typically for 6 weeks postoperatively. Range-of-motion exercises typically are started once the fixator is removed, but non–weight bearing is recommended for 12 weeks postoperatively with these injuries.

NAVICULAR INJURIES

Navicular fractures typically are associated with high-energy crushing or axial-load mechanisms, frequently with an abduction and flexion component.[7] Radiographic images typically underestimate the extent of injury, making CT evaluation mandatory when navicular injury is suspected. Sangeorzan and colleagues[8] devised a classification system that categorizes displaced tarsal navicular body fractures that categorizes the fractures into three types with severity increasing from type one to type three. With increasing severity of the injury, it proved more difficult to obtain a satisfactory reduction. In their series, operative treatment proved difficult, and satisfactory results were achieved in less than 50% of type three injuries.[8] Anatomic reduction is crucial to the outcome of navicular fractures. At a minimum, 60% of the articular surface of the navicular is required to prevent talonavicular instability and subluxation after healing.[9]

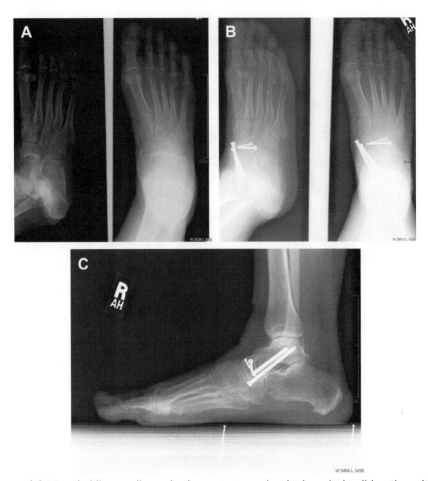

Fig. 2. (*A*) AP and oblique radiographs demonstrate a missed talonavicular dislocation with lateral dislocation of the talar head sustained in an MVA. Note the large impaction of the talar head. The injury was not identified until 7 weeks after it occurred. (*B, C*) Treatment consisted of primary arthrodesis of the talonavicular joint after reduction.

Adduction through the midfoot can be seen as a deformity from medial column shortening. Talonavicular motion lost though trauma or subsequent arthrodesis restricts overall hindfoot motion[5] and decreases subtalar motion by approximately 80%.[10] Long-term problems can arise from altered hindfoot kinematics as a result of arthrodesis. Every effort should be made to preserve the integrity of this joint for as long as possible. Posttraumatic arthrosis at the talonavicular joint is well documented as the most common complication after navicular fractures.[11] Patients typically present with decreased range of motion and pain, which often is worse on uneven surfaces. As in other articular fractures, a strong correlation has been found between the reduction quality of the navicular articular surface and the subsequent development of posttraumatic arthrosis.[8]

The navicular blood supply is circumferential in nature. A large anastomotic network is formed via branches of the dorsalis pedis and medial plantar arteries. The radial

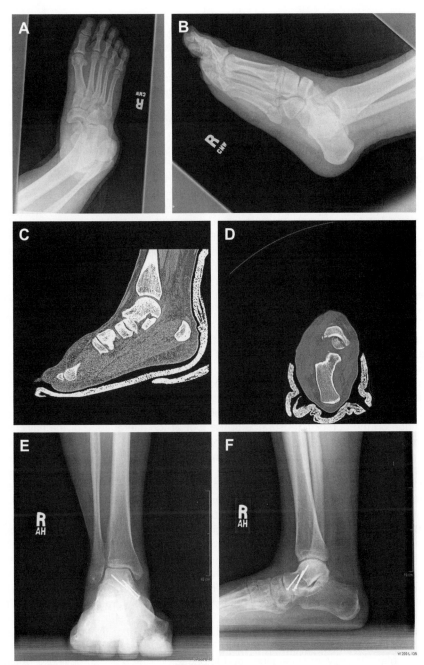

Fig. 3. (*A*) AP and (*B*) lateral radiographs demonstrate a talar head fracture with associated pantalar dislocation. (*C*) Sagital and (*D*) axial CT images show the talar head to be turned 180 degrees. The injury was treated with distraction to reduce the talar head articular fragment and (*E, F*) open reduction and internal fixation. A spanning external fixator was left on for six weeks because of instability at the ankle and subtalar joints.

nature of the vascular complex results in a relatively hypovascular area in the central portion of the navicular bone.[12] The surgeon is presented with the significant challenge of weighing surgical exposure against the preservation of an already tenuous blood supply. Avascular necrosis or non-union can occur from excessive soft tissue stripping at the time of fixation.

Because of the poor blood supply and the key role of the navicular in hindfoot function, all fractures with any displacement should be treated operatively. Without reconstruction, late deformity can occur as the talar head migrates into the fracture plane (**Fig. 4**). Simple fracture patterns can be treated with lag screw fixation. Small incisions can be made for the insertion of a reduction clamp, and fixation can be achieved with 2.7- or 2.4-mm screws. If comminution is present, lag fixation should be avoided to prevent narrowing the concavity of the articular surface of the navicular.

More comminuted injuries require more advanced fixation techniques. Typically, some form of distraction is required to allow visualization of the navicular and its proximal and distal articulations. This distraction can be achieved using a large external fixator, which typically is placed at the time of initial injury and consists of pins in the first metatarsal, a transcalcaneal pin, and a pin into the fourth and fifth metatarsals. Distraction should be applied both medially and laterally, allowing the length of both columns to be restored. Through distraction, the talar head is disimpacted from the central portion of the navicular, creating room for the reduction of the navicular fragments.

Two incisions are used in more comminuted injuries to allow visualization of a greater percentage of the articular surface and more accurate reconstruction as well as more options for the placement of fixation. A medial incision is placed in the interval between the anterior tibialis and posterior tibialis tendons. The talonavicular and naviculocuneiform joints are visualized through arthrotomies made vertically to avoid soft tissue stripping to the medial aspect of the navicular and to maintain vascularity to the navicular. The second incision, guided by intraoperative fluoroscopy, is made on the dorsolateral surface of the foot at the lateral edge of the navicular. Care must be taken to avoid injury to the superficial peroneal nerve during dissection. Provisional fixation is achieved with Kirschner wires, which also can be used to manipulate small fragments into position.

Definitive fixation consists of screws for less comminuted injuries. In more severe injuries a mini fragment plate may be contoured and passed under the dorsal soft tissues. Initially this technique was described using a five-hole plate with a curve of 120° (the cross section of one third of a circular tube) that was bent slightly, placed subcutaneously, and held in place by two to four 4.0-mm cortical screws.[13] The plate acts as a buttress to prevent dorsal extrusion of fracture fragments as a result of comminution. A mini fragment T plate works well for this purpose. The "T" portion of the plate is used on the more comminuted side of the navicular (**Fig. 5**). The ability to place more screws allows better control of smaller fracture fragments. The articular reduction is confirmed by direct visualization of the articular surfaces, palpation, and fluoroscopic imaging. Distraction is reduced after fixation is completed. In cases of severe comminution, the surgeon may consider leaving the external fixator in place to prevent subsidence and impaction of the reduced navicular. Atraumatic suture techniques are used for closure, and a well-padded splint is applied. If the external fixator is left in place, it is removed 6 weeks postoperatively, at which time range-of-motion exercise is initiated. Typically, non–weight-bearing status is maintained for 12 weeks after surgery. Outcomes measures for mini fragment plate fixation for highly comminuted navicular fractures are being evaluated at Sparrow Health System, and early results are encouraging.

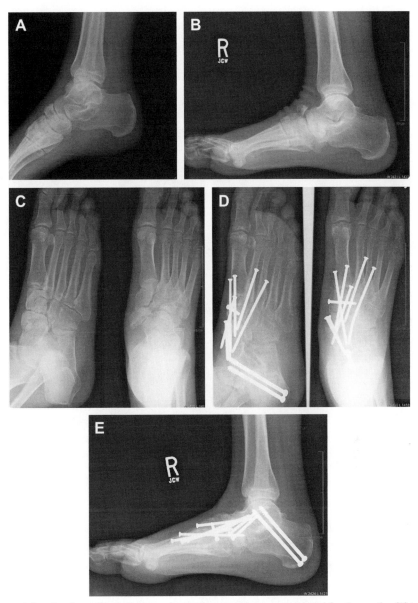

Fig. 4. (*A*) A simple navicular fracture in a college professor was missed for 3 months. (*B*) Lateral (*C*) AP and oblique radiographs demonstrate distal·migration of the talar head through the navicular defect. (*D*) The injury was treated surgically with arthrodesis. (*E*) The subtalar joint also was fused because the patient had a history of insulin-dependent diabetes.

CUNEIFORM FRACTURES

Fractures of the cuneiforms rarely occur in isolation. Most often they occur as part of a more complex injury with other associated fractures and or dislocations through the talonavicular, cuboid, or tarsometatarsal joints. They result from a significant abductive or adductive force on the forefoot or from a direct crushing or axial injury.

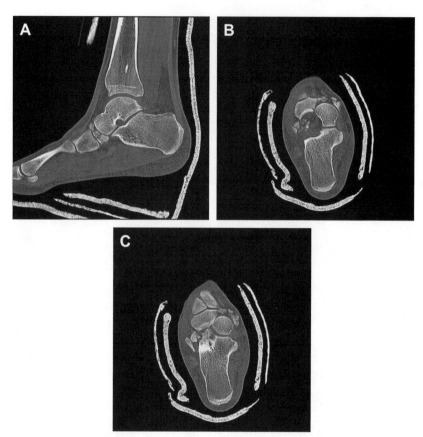

Fig. 5. An intoxicated man drove into a tree and sustained injuries including severe deformity at Chopart's joints as demonstrated on (*A*) coronal and (*B, C*) axial CT images. A fixator was applied for distraction at time of presentation. (*D, E*) The patient underwent open reduction and internal fixation of the cuboid and navicular when soft tissues permitted.

Isolated nondisplaced fractures may be treated with cast immobilization and non–weight bearing.

Displaced fractures should be treated with operative fixation to preserve the integrity of both the longitudinal and transverse arch. This fixation can be accomplished by lag screw fixation in simple fractures with no comminution. In more comminuted injuries fixation may span into noninjured cuneiforms. Longitudinal screws extending from the metatarsal bases into the navicular also may be used to provide additional stability. If severe comminution is present, bridge plating can be used to maintain medial column length and can extend from the first metatarsal base to the navicular or talus as necessary (**Fig. 6**).[14] Plates that span the talonavicular joint are removed after healing has occurred. Alternatively, plating can be performed on the dorsum of the foot and extend from the base of the metatarsal to the navicular. Mini fragment or locked mini fragment plates typically are used in this location (**Fig. 7**). Other associated injuries to the foot should be treated appropriately.

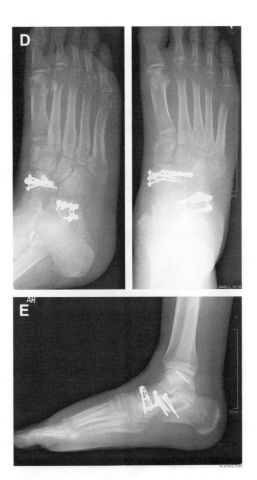

Fig. 5. *(continued)*

Lateral Column Injuries

Cuboid fractures

The cuboid is saddle shaped and articulates proximally with the calcaneus and distally with the fourth and fifth metatarsals. The dorsal calcaneocuboid, cuneocuboid, cubonavicular, and cubometatarsal ligaments envelope the dorsal surface. The deep fibers of the long plantar ligament attach to the proximal portion of the plantar ridge. A "slip" of the tibialis posterior and flexor hallucis brevis attach to the proximal-medial portion of the cuboid. A tuberosity on the plantar surface of the bone serves as an attachment for the plantar ligament. This ligament, which also gives off attachments to the calcaneus and the second, third, fourth, and possibly fifth metatarsals, is integral in maintaining the lateral longitudinal arch of the midfoot.[15]

The major source of blood supply to the dorsum of the cuboid is from the anterior tibial artery. The anterior tibial artery continues as the dorsalis pedis artery and gives off the proximal lateral tarsal artery at about the level of the talar neck. The transverse pedicle branch arises from this artery and supplies the major nutrient vessels to the cuboid.[16]

The cuboid plays an important role in maintaining the lateral column of the foot and must work in concert with the periarticular ligaments and osseous structures surrounding it for normal gait to occur. Cuboid fractures rarely present as an isolated

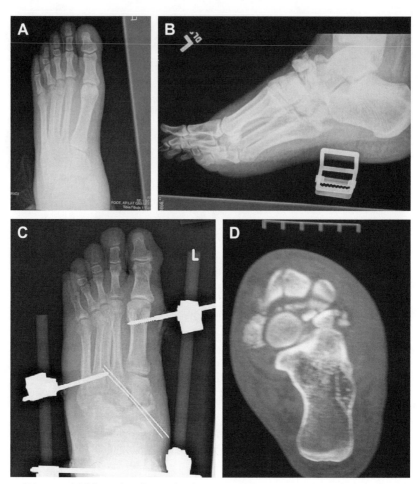

Fig. 6. (A) AP and (B) lateral radiographs demonstrate a severe crushing injury of navicular, cuboid, and all cuneiforms. (C) The injury was initially treated with an external fixator followed by delayed open reduction and fixation and bridge plating when soft tissues permitted. (D) Axial CT scan demonstrates extensive comminution of the Chopart joints. (E, F) The plate was left in long term because it did not cross talonavicular joint.

injury and generally are caused by lower-energy mechanisms of injury. Cuboid fractures that are stable and nondisplaced usually can be managed nonoperatively. Simple fracture patterns may be treated with 6 to 8 weeks of non–weight bearing.

More complex injuries usually are the result of a crushing injury, as seen in MVAs. They result from a global shortening of the midfoot through both the medial and lateral columns or as a result of a severe abduction force to the forefoot. This force produces a severely comminuted fracture caused by the cuboid being crushed between the fourth and fifth metatarsal bases and the anterior process of the calcaneus, as if by a nutcracker. The foot usually is in a position of plantar flexion and/or abduction.[17] Weber and Locher[18] reported on the reconstruction of 12 cuboid compression fractures, 10 of which were associated with another midfoot fracture. Eleven of the 12 fractures were consistent with a "nutcracker"-type fracture.[19] If a patient is found to have

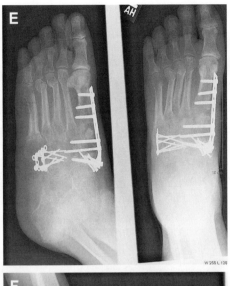

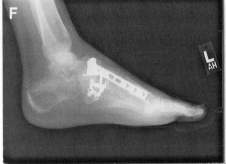

Fig. 6. (*continued*)

a cuboid fracture consistent with compression of the lateral column, it is necessary to rule out injury/fracture of the medial column.

Standard anteroposterior, lateral, and oblique radiographs of the involved foot should be obtained. The cuboid is best visualized best radiographically on the oblique radiograph. When there is a high index of suspicion for injury but no obvious fracture, stress radiographs may be valuable. A CT scan may help delineate bony damage and visualize articular step-off that may not be apparent on conventional radiographs.

The goals of surgical intervention should include re-establishing length to the lateral column and anatomic restoration and stable fixation of the articular surfaces. In more comminuted fractures articular incongruity is present at one or both joints. The cuboid itself is significantly shortened, shortening the lateral column as a whole. Distraction can be achieved by using an external fixation device, allowing disimpaction of the cuboid, restoration of the overall length, and improved visualization of both the calcaneocuboid and cuboid-metatarsal articulations. Bone-specific plates are available and allow grafting of both articular surfaces (**Fig. 8**). Often bone grafting of the central void of the cuboid is necessary and can be accomplished with cancellous bone. Sangeorzan and Swiontkowski[20] reported good functional results in four cases of

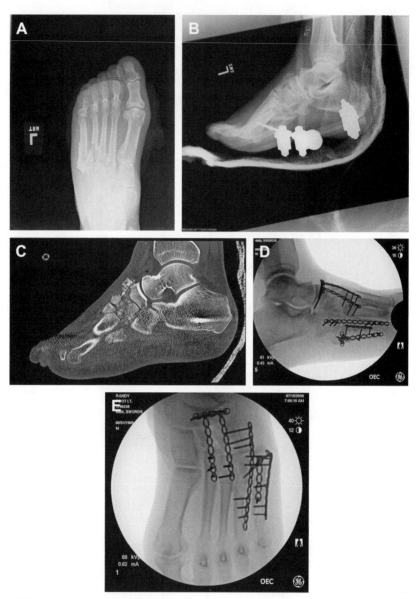

Fig. 7. (*A*) Severe injury to cuneiforms occurred from a gunshot wound through the midfoot. (*B*) The injury was treated with delayed fixation consisting of (*C*) bridge plating dorsally from (*D*) the metatarsal bases to (*E*) the navicular.

cuboid fractures that were treated with open reduction and internal fixation using iliac crest bone graft when needed for restoration of length.

Operative reconstruction of displaced cuboid fractures is necessary, because post-traumatic shortening of the lateral column of the foot is poorly tolerated, and persistent incongruity of the joint surfaces can lead to painful arthrosis. The calcaneocuboid and cuboid-metatarsal articulations are considered essential joints, because of the amount of inherent motion needed to accommodate to nonlevel terrain. Therefore

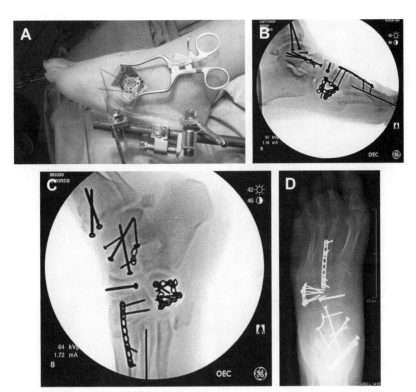

Fig. 8. A highly comminuted cuboid fracture that occurred in an MVA. (*A*) Note the cuboid plate on bone with distractor present to assist with (*B, C*) reduction and visualization of articular surfaces. (*D*) The fifth metatarsal was lost as a result of the trauma.

posttraumatic arthrosis in the calcaneocuboid and cuboid-metatarsal articulations is poorly tolerated. Because there is no reliable salvage procedure for posttraumatic arthrosis in these articulations, every effort should be made to restore articular congruity anatomically at the time of fixation.

Anterior process calcaneus fractures

Occasionally, the cuboid does not fracture with the abduction force, but the anterior process of the calcaneus does. This situation typically occurs with an impaction injury of the articular surface, resulting in shortening of the lateral column. This fracture is treated like a cuboid fracture. Distraction through an external fixator, articular disimpaction/reconstruction, and supportive bone grafting are the hallmarks of surgical treatment (**Fig. 9**).

OUTCOMES

Two major outcome studies provide insight into these injuries. In a review of 100 patients who had 110 Chopart injuries, better outcomes were seen in individuals treated with open reduction and operative fixation, which allows the most accurate reconstruction of osseous anatomy.[21] Isolated fractures of the midfoot, Chopart injuries, and Lisfranc injuries had similar outcome scores as determined by the American Orthopaedic Foot and Ankle Society score and the Hannover Scoring System. Combined Chopart-Lisfranc injuries had significantly lower scores. Variations in age,

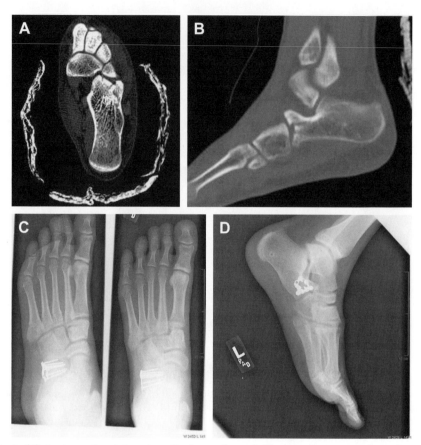

Fig. 9. (*A*) An impaction injury to articular surface of (*B*) the calcaneus at the calcaneal cuboid joint. (*C*) The injury was treated with elevation of articular surface and (*D*) bone grafting.

gender, cause of injury, and time to treatment did not affect outcome scores significantly. A correlation was seen between correct medial and lateral column lengths and good functional results.[22]

For best results these injuries should be recognized early. Formal open fixation with restoration of anatomy should be undertaken when soft tissue swelling allows. The best possible outcomes can be achieved by restoring normal alignment of both medial and lateral columns, restoring articular congruity, and maintaining reduction over time. These injuries are severe. Despite best efforts at reconstruction, posttraumatic arthritis will occur in some cases. Patients who have these injuries should be counseled about potential complications and long-term functional impairment from these injuries.

REFERENCES

1. Klaue K. Chopart fractures. Injury 2004;35:SB64–70.
2. Richter M, Wippermann B, Thermann H, et al. Plantar impact causing midfoot fractures result in higher forces in Chopart's joint than in the ankle joint. J Orthop Res 2002;20:222–32.

3. Wilson LS, Mizel MS, Michelson JD. Foot and ankle injuries in motor vehicle accidents. Foot Ankle Int 2001;22(8):649–52.
4. De Asla RJ, Deland JT. Anatomy and biomechanics of the foot and ankle. In: Thoradson DB, editor. Orthopaedic surgery essentials foot and ankle. Philadelphia: Lippincott Williams & Wilkins; 2004. p. 1–23.
5. Astion DJ, Deland JT, Otis JC, et al. Motion of the hindfoot after simulated arthrodesis. J Bone Joint Surg [Am] 1997;79:241–6.
6. Hansen ST. Functional reconstruction of the foot and ankle. Philadelphia: Lippencott, Williams and Wilkins; 2000.
7. Eichenholtz SN, Levine DB. Fractures of the tarsal navicular bone. Clin Orthop 1964;34:142–57.
8. Sangeorzan BJ, Benirschke SK, Mosca V, et al. Displaced intraarticular fractures of the tarsal navicular. J Bone Joint Surg [Am] 1989;71:1504–10.
9. Pinney SJ, Sangeorzan BJ. Fractures of the tarsal bones. Orthop Clin North Am 2001;32:21–33.
10. Walker N, Stukenborg C, Savory KM, et al. Hindfoot motion after isolated and combined arthrodeses: measurements in anatomic specimens. Foot Ankle Int 2000;21:921–7.
11. Thordarson DB. Fractures of the midfoot and forefoot. In: Myerson MS, editor. Foot and ankle disorders. Philadelphia: WB Saunders; 2000. p. 1265–96.
12. Torg J, Pavlov H, Cooley L, et al. Stress fractures of the tarsal navicular: a retrospective review of twenty-one cases. J Bone Joint Surg [Am] 1982;64:700–12.
13. Cammack PM, Donahue MP, Manoli A. The bridge and barrel hoop plates as alternatives to external fixation techniques in the foot and ankle. Foot Ankle Clin 2004;9:625–35.
14. Schildhauer TA, Nork SE, Sangeorzan BJ. Temporary bridge plating of the medial column in severe midfoot injuries. J Orthop Trauma 2003;17(7):513–20.
15. Sarrafian SK. Anatomy of the foot and ankle. 2nd edition. Philadelphia: JB Lippincott; 1993. p. 8–18, 294–339.
16. Gilbert BJ, Horst F, Nunley JA. Potential donor rotational bone grafts using vascular territories in the foot and ankle. J Bone Joint Surg [Am] 2004;86:1857–73.
17. Miller CM, Winter WG, Bucknell AI, et al. Injuries to the midtarsal joint and lesser tarsal bones. J Am Acad Orthop Surg 1998;6:249–58.
18. Weber M, Locher S. Reconstruction of the cuboid in compression fractures: short to midterm results in 12 patients. Foot Ankle Int 2002;23(11):1108–1013.
19. Hermel MB, Gershon-Cohen J. Nutcracker fracture of the cuboid by indirect violence. Radiology 1953;60:850–4.
20. Sangeorzan BJ, Swiontkowski MF. Displaced fractures of the cuboid. J Bone Joint Surg [Br] 1990;72:376–8.
21. Richter M, Thermann F, Huefner T, et al. Chopart joint fracture-dislocation: initial open reduction provides better outcome than closed reduction. Foot Ankle Int 2004;25(5):340–8.
22. Richter M, Wippermann B, Krettek C, et al. Fractures and fracture dislocations of the midfoot: occurrence, causes and long-term results. Foot Ankle Int 2001;22(5): 392–8.

Making Sense of Lisfranc Injuries

J. Chris Coetzee, MD

KEYWORDS

- Lisfranc injuries • Midfoot sprains • Classification
- Management

Management of Lisfranc injuries has evoked significant debate and controversy over the years, and there is no indication that the controversy is nearing an end. Probably the main reason for the controversy is because a "Lisfranc Injury" is part of a very wide and poorly defined spectrum of injuries. Not all Lisfranc injuries are created equal, and there will never be a single treatment option for all these injuries. Lisfranc injuries are relatively uncommon, but if undetected, untreated or under-treated can cause morbidity and disability. The objective of this article is to provide guidelines for treatment of the spectrum of Lisfranc injuries.

ANATOMY

The unique anatomy of the Lisfranc joints contributes to the spectrum of injury patterns. The stability of the tarsometatarsal (TMT) joint complex is maintained by a combination of the wedge-shaped configuration of the metatarsal bases and their corresponding cuneiform articulations, as well as the ligamentous support.

Structurally, the midfoot can be divided into columns: the medial column consists of the first metatarsal, medial cuneiform, and its navicular facet; the middle column consists of the second and third metatarsals, their corresponding cuneiforms, and the central and lateral facets of the navicular; the lateral column consists of the fourth and fifth metatarsals and their articulations with the cuboid. The second metatarsal is recessed as a keystone between the medial and lateral cuneiforms and the addition of the strong plantar ligaments "lock" the metatarsals to the midfoot. Lisfranc's ligament is composed of three portions running from the medial cuneiform to the base of the second metatarsal. The strongest part is the plantar portion of the ligament, which is the main stabilizing component of the first and second metatarsal interspace. There are 5 to 10 degrees at the first TMT joint, minimal motion at the second and third TMT joints, and 10 to 20 degrees at the fourth and fifth metatarsal-cuboid, which is important in accommodating uneven ground.

Department of Orthopedics, University of Minnesota, 775 Prairie Center Drive, #250, Eden Prairie, MN 55344, USA
E-mail address: jcc@ocpamn.com

Foot Ankle Clin N Am 13 (2008) 695–704
doi:10.1016/j.fcl.2008.07.001
1083-7515/08/$ – see front matter © 2008 Elsevier Inc. All rights reserved.

foot.theclinics.com

An important factor to remember is that the Lisfranc joints have little inherent stability. The joints are oriented as flat on flat surfaces and rely on ligamentous stability to maintain reduction such that without ligamentous stability the "arch" will collapse (**Fig. 1**A, B).

MECHANISM OF INJURY

Injuries to the TMT joints can be caused by direct or indirect forces. Myerson and colleagues[1] showed that with direct injuries the direction of displacement is dependent on the point of application of the injuring force. The direct force/axial load usually centers on the dorsum of the foot, which creates a tensile force on the plantar side of the TMT joints, and if torn, the Lisfranc complex becomes unstable. The intensity and angle of the force will determine whether there are fractures and/or ligamentous injuries.

Indirect forces are more common and include bending or twisting moments applied to the midfoot, such as a football player being struck from behind with the involved ankle and foot in a hyperplantarflexed position. The history and mechanism may help to determine the severity, stability, and prognosis of the injury. The injury pattern may be a "benign" or partial sprain, whereby only the dorsal intertarsal ligaments are torn and the strong plantar ligaments remain intact; in this instance, there is no widening of the intermetatarsal space, and return to activity is regulated by pain and discomfort. With higher energy patterns, the strong plantar ligaments are also torn, making the TMT complex very unstable, and in which case the metatarsals usually dislocate dorsally.

CLASSIFICATION

There is considerable difficulty in attempting to accurately group Lisfranc injuries into neatly organized compartments because of the multiple variations and levels of severity in the injury complex. The classification by Hardcastle and colleagues[2] is based on the three-column concept of the midfoot and includes type A as a total incongruity; type B as a partial incongruity; and type C as a divergent incongruity. The importance of this classification is that injury to one portion of a column usually indicates injury to other portions of that column.[3] Myerson and colleagues[1] proposed a more complete

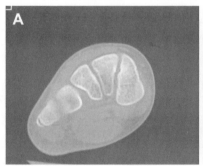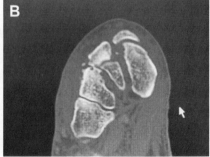

Fig. 1. (*A*) The TMT joints form the transverse arch of the foot. With the unique boney configuration, with "flat on flat" joints, the stability is almost exclusively dependent on the strong ligamentous support. (*B*) With disruption of the ligamentous structures there is no inherent stability in the Lisfranc complex, and it should be obvious that the bone will separate and displace with weight bearing.

classification system by subdividing the Hardcastle types into B1, B2, C1, and C2 depending on the complexity of the injury.

Nunley and Vertullo[4] introduced a useful classification for subtle Lisfranc injuries with minimal or no displacement on weight-bearing films. Stage 1 is an injury in which the patient is able to bear weight, but not return to previous activity; there is point tenderness over the TMT joint and weight-bearing radiographs show less than 2-mm diastasis between the first and second rays and no collapse of the medial arch. Stage 2 has similar clinical findings, but there is more than 2- to 5-mm diastasis on radiographs, with no arch collapse on lateral view. Stage 3 has more than 2- to 5-mm diastasis radiographically with collapse of the longitudinal arch collapse.[4]

CLINICAL PICTURE

Patients with a Lisfranc almost universally present with pain and swelling in the mid-foot and difficulty bearing weight. Plantar ecchymosis indicates significant soft tissue disruption, and is suggestive of a Lisfranc injury until proven otherwise, even if the plain radiographs do not show any fractures.

IMAGING AND CLINICAL CONFIRMATION

Weight bearing (as much as tolerated) anteroposterior (AP), oblique, and lateral radiographs of the foot are indicated in the event of a suspected Lisfranc injury, and should include both feet as a comparative study. If weight-bearing radiographs are normal but there remains a strong suspicion of a Lisfranc injury, one should consider a CT scan, loaded if possible. MRI can also be helpful in determining the extent of ligamentous involvement in a "subtle" injury; however, an examination under anesthesia might ultimately be the most reliable way to evaluate the extent of instability in the absence of fractures.

TREATMENT

Because of the marked variability in pathoanatomy, treatment of Lisfranc injuries should be individualized to the actual injury pattern and extent of instability: with a partial ligamentous disruption (hyperplantarflexion injury) and stable weight-bearing radiographs, only symptomatic treatment is required; conversely, with a severely comminuted fracture-dislocation with extensive joint damage, open reduction and internal fixation will most certainly be required, and may even further benefit from a primary arthrodesis.

For treatment purposes, Lisfranc injuries should be divided into two major groups: incomplete ligamentous disruption and complete ligamentous disruption. Both groups can include any variation of transverse and/or longitudinal injury patterns.

- Incomplete ligamentous disruption
  a. Stage 1: less than 2 mm diastases. No arch collapse.
  b. Stage 2: >2–5 mm diastases. No arch collapse.
  c. Stage 3: >2–5 mm diastases. Medial longitudinal arch collapse.
- Complete ligamentous disruption
  a. Without significant intra-articular fractures.
  b. With significant intra-articular comminution.

Incomplete Ligamentous Disruption

There is little controversy with respect to management in this group. In Stages 1 and 2 the plantar ligaments are intact, which is always prognostically favorable. Stage 1 injuries can usually be treated nonoperatively; stage 2 and 3 injuries will need a closed or open reduction and internal fixation.[4,5] The fixation construct should address all the elements of the instability, whether localized to the tarsometatarsal joints alone, or any combination of intercuneiform and cuneiform-navicular joints. There is adequate proof in the literature that an anatomic reduction and stable fixation will lead to the highest satisfaction rate.[1,6–9]

The following algorithm is suggested (**Fig. 2**A–D).

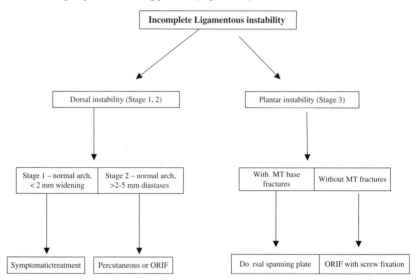

Traditional open reduction, internal fixation (ORIF) techniques consist of 3.5-mm cortical screws in noncompression mode; in the event of significant metatarsal comminution, low-profile bridge plating across the involved joints is indicated to maintain alignment and length while the fractures and joints heal.[10] The lateral metatarsal-cuboid joints usually reduce with reduction of the medial three rays; if there is still an appreciable instability, the lateral rays are reduced and immobilized with percutaneus Kirschner wires (K-wires).

Complete Ligamentous Disruption

The true controversy in the Lisfranc injury spectrum is in patients with complete ligamentous instability (**Fig. 3**A–I). In patterns with intra-articular extension, particularly those with one or two big fragments and typically at the second metatarsal base, conventional ORIF is probably warranted, especially if there is a large plantar-medial fragment at the second metatarsal base and the remainder of the metatarsal is dislocated dorsally. In this instance, the Lisfranc ligament may still be intact and attached to the plantar medial fragment, such that traditional ORIF will render the entire construct stable. In the event of multiple joint fragments, however, it is unlikely that one will be able to adequately reconstruct the joint without subsequent early degeneration of the joint; a primary fusion may therefore be the best option to maximize function in this group.

Patients with minimal or no fractures, but completely dislocated joints, create the biggest therapeutic challenge. Currently the recommended and accepted treatment

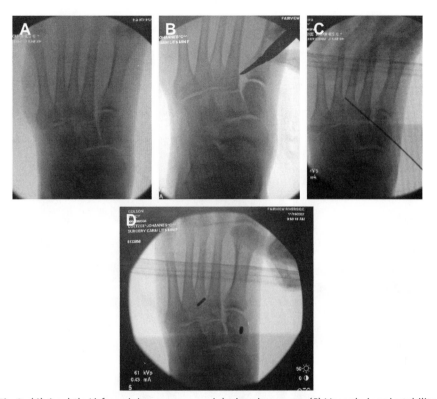

Fig. 2. (A) A subtle Lisfranc injury on non–weight-bearing x-rays. (B) Very obvious instability between the first and second rays with a disrupted Lisfranc ligament. There was no longitudinal instability and the plantar ligaments were intact. (C) Because of the localized instability, it was possible to use a simple fixation technique. (D) Tightrope fixation of an isolated Lisfranc instability with good long-term result.

of Lisfranc complex injuries is ORIF.[1,6–8,11,12] Unfortunately, despite appropriate initial treatment, some patients may go on to posttraumatic arthritis—the reported incidence of osteoarthritis after ORIF of Lisfranc dislocations is 40% to 94%.[1,7,8,11–13] These patients often require a conversion to an arthrodesis of the TMT joints.

Historic articles on the management of Lisfranc injuries should be read with due diligence. Most, if not all, studies are retrospective, and report "good to excellent" results in most patients, with brief mention that a certain percentage will go on to develop degenerative changes. Very few articles however mention what outcomes criteria were used to determine good or excellent. Could they return to their previous level of activity? Including sporting activities? How much pain, etc? I will dare to say that most TMT dislocations treated with **temporary** fixation, whether screws, plates, or K-wires, will eventually develop degenerative joint disease (DJD) and collapse. As previously discussed, the flat on flat joint configuration offers no inherent stability such that in the event of a complete ligamentous disruption, the natural forces over the joints will eventually cause the medial longitudinal arch to collapse and the foot will also drift into abduction. Part of the controversy in these severe Lisfranc injuries is whether or not to remove the screws after an ORIF. If you believe the screws should not be removed, how does it differ from a fusion?

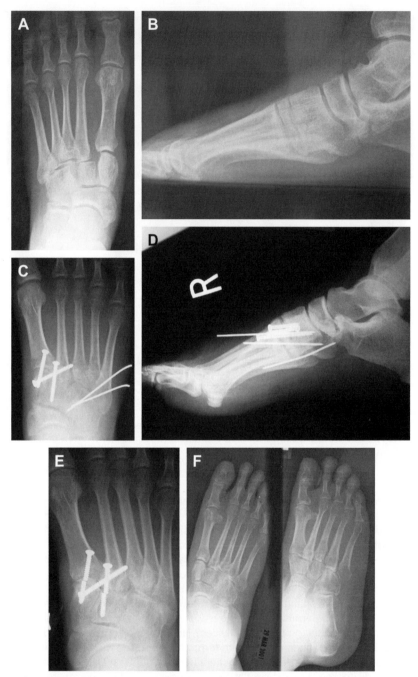

Fig. 3. (*A, B*) The weight-bearing AP and lateral of an incomplete ligamentous disruption (stage 3). (*C, D*) A conventional ORIF. (*E*) Six-month x-ray shows breakage of the screws. (*F*) After removal of the screws, there are already signs of early DJD and collapse of the mid-foot. (*G*) Four years later there is severe DJD and deformity of the tarsometatarsal joints. (*H, I*) Subsequent fusion of the Lisfranc joint 4 years and 6 months after the index injury.

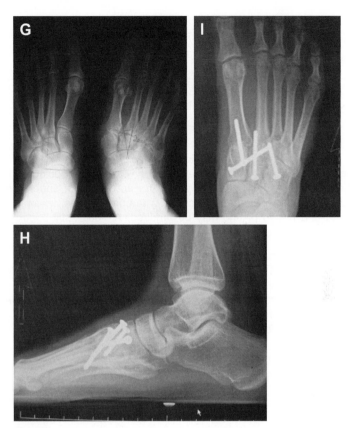

Fig. 3. (continued)

Ly and Coetzee[13] showed that patients treated with primary arthrodeses did better at every time interval than those treated with ORIF with respect to previous level of activity (**Table 1**). Vertullo and Nunley[14] also reported on five professional athletes, including two National Football League (NFL) players who returned to the NFL after Lisfranc fusions. As part of their study, they conducted a questionnaire to foot and ankle surgeons regarding expected return to activity following arthrodesis in the foot and ankle: almost 100% felt that an athlete could return to golf, skiing, or tennis; 76% felt it should be no problem to jog, but only 54% felt that return to sprinting would be possible; between 62% and 69% felt that an athlete could return to professional football, soccer, or basketball. There is unfortunately no reported literature on the percentage of athletes who will be able to return after an ORIF of the Lisfranc joints.

In our study, the reoperation rate in the ORIF group was 75%, which included hardware removals and conversions to fusions; the reoperation rate in the fusion group was 20%.[13] This is very similar to the reoperation rate reported by Anderson and colleagues,[15] in a prospective randomized study, showing reoperation rates of 79% in the ORIF group and 17% in the fusion group, respectively. An interesting observation since our study[13] is that at least 50% of the patients with an ORIF for a complete dislocation find it hard, if not impossible to do multiple single-leg heel raises, while the arthrodeses group has no problems with that.

Table 1
Clinical questionnaire

Percentage Level of Participation Compared with Pre-Injury Status	6 Month, %	12 Month, %	24 Month, %
Fusion	62	86	92
Open reduction, internal fixation (ORIF)	44	61	65

To do a primary fusion is no more difficult than an ORIF. If the bone structure is well maintained, the joints are prepared by removing the cartilage, reducing the joints, and placing the screws exactly the same way as for an ORIF, but under compression (**Fig. 4**A, B). In cases of significant fractures with comminution, screw fixation may be precluded and bridge plating may be required. Although still controversial, the following approach is suggested.

- Indications for primary fusions of Lisfranc fractures and dislocations
  1) Major ligamentous disruptions with multidirectional instability/dislocation of the Lisfranc joints.
  2) Comminuted intra-articular fractures at the base of the first or second metatarsal
  3) Crush injuries of the midfoot with intra-articular fracture dislocation
- Contraindications for primary fusions for Lisfranc injuries
  1) Lisfranc injuries in children with open physes
  2) Incomplete ligamentous injuries (see previous list)
  3) Unidirectional Lisfranc instability
  4) Unstable extra-articular metatarsal bases fractures with questionable ligamentous disruption

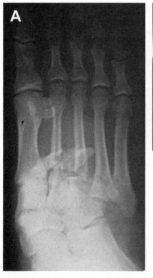
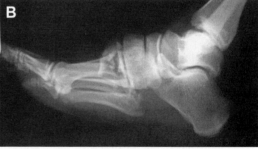

Fig. 4. (*A, B*) Severely comminuted, intra-articular fracture dislocation of the TMT joints. There should be very little controversy that the best option here is a primary fusion.

We agree with Kuo and colleagues[12] that the purely ligamentous Lisfranc injuries do not always heal with ORIF. They reported that there was a tendency for this type of injury to have an increased prevalence of osteoarthrosis (6 of 15 patients or 40%). Mulier and colleagues[11] performed a surgeon-randomized study on 28 patients with Lisfranc dislocations. They compared ORIF (16 patients) to complete arthrodesis (6 patients) and partial arthrodesis (6 patients), and at final follow-up (30 months) 94% of the ORIF group already had degenerative changes of the TMT joints on radiographs. Although all such patients are not likely become symptomatic enough to fuse, it seems intuitive that a high percentage will be limited in function to some degree—indeed, 12% of their ORIF group needed a conversion to a fusion within 14 months.[11]

There have been several recent articles regarding complete versus partial arthrodesis for Lisfranc injuries.[9,13,15] The consensus is that only the medial two to three rays should be fused. We concur with Komenda and colleagues[16] and Sangeorzan and colleagues[7] that it is favorable to preserve motion in the lateral two rays and that it is not necessary to do a complete fusion to obtain optimum results. Komenda and colleagues[16] reported the results of late arthrodesis on posttraumatic tarsometatarsal joint injury at a mean of 35 months after the injury; their mean postoperative American Orthopaedic Foot and Ankle Society Midfoot Score was 78 with a mean follow-up of 50 months. There is increasing evidence to suggest that in severe injuries, a primary fusion may allow patients to avoid persistent pain and disability from posttraumatic arthritis.

SUMMARY

There is no single correct way of treating all Lisfranc injuries. The incomplete ligamentous disruption group will vary from subtle, nondisplaced injuries that need activity modification only, to partially unstable injuries that need an ORIF. An anatomic reduction and stable fixation is advocated. If the screws are removed, it should not be done before 6 months. The complete dislocations, with or without fracture, are more difficult to treat. The insult of the injury predisposes this group to inferior long-term results. A high percentage of them will eventually go on to develop DJD. It is true that not all of them will be symptomatic enough to warrant a fusion, but at this point in time there is no way to determine who will do well and who not.

There are a few current prospective randomized studies under way comparing primary arthrodeses to ORIF in this completely unstable group. The results so far show that a primary fusion for a completely dislocated Lisfranc injury does better at every interval, has fewer complications, and a lower reoperation rate than a standard ORIF.

This does not mean every Lisfranc injury needs a fusion. This article gives the author's approach to treating Lisfranc injuries that shows a smaller subset of injuries will be treated with a primary fusion. If it is felt that a fusion is the correct choice for a specific injury pattern, it is currently done irrespective of the patient's level of sporting activity. As long as everyone involved realizes that a very severe injury occurred and that the foot "will never be the same," a fusion in a select group of injuries does better than if a formal ORIF would have been done.

REFERENCES

1. Myerson MS, Fisher RT, Burgess AR, et al. Fracture dislocations of the tarsometatarsal joints: end results correlated with pathology and treatment. Foot Ankle 1986;6(5):225–42.

2. Hardcastle PH, Reschauer R, Kutscha-Lissberg E, et al. Injuries to the tarsometa-tarsal joint. Incidence, classification and treatment. J Bone Joint Surg Br 1982; 64(3):349–56.

3. Talarico RH, Hamilton GA, Ford LA, et al. Fracture dislocations of the tarsometa-tarsal joints: analysis of interrater reliability in using the modified Hardcastle clas-sification system. J Foot Ankle Surg 2006;45(5):300–3.

4. Nunley JA, Vertullo CJ. Classification, investigation, and management of midfoot sprains: Lisfranc injuries in athletes. Am J Sports Med 2002;30:871–8.

5. Lattermann C, Goldstein JL, Wukich DK, et al. Practical management of Lisfranc injuries in athletes. Clin J Sport Med 2007;17(4):311–5.

6. Arntz CR, Veith RG, Hansen ST. Fractures and fracture-dislocations of the tarso-metatarsal joint. J Bone Joint Surg Am 1988;70:173–81.

7. Sangeorzan BJ, Veith RG, Hansen ST. Salvage of Lisfranc's tarsometatarsal joint by arthrodesis. Foot Ankle 1990;10:193–200.

8. Arntz CT, Hansen ST. Dislocation and fracture dislocations of the tarsometarsal joints. Orthop Clin North Am 1987;18:105–14.

9. Lee CA, Birkedal JP, Dickerson EA, et al. Stabilization of Lisfranc joint injuries: a biomechanical study. Foot Ankle Int 2004;25(5):365–70.

10. Alberta FG, Aronow MS, Barrero M, et al. Ligamentous Lisfranc joint injuries: a bio-mechanical comparison of dorsal plate and transarticular screw fixation. Foot Ankle Int 2005;26(6):462–73.

11. Mulier T, Reynders P, Dereymaeker G, et al. Severe Lisfrancs injuries: Primary arthrodesis or ORIF? Foot Ankle Int 2002;23:902–5.

12. Kuo RS, Tejwani NC, DiGiovanni CW, et al. Outcome after open reduction and in-ternal fixation of Lisfranc joint injuries. J Bone Joint Surg Am 2000;82:1609–18.

13. Ly TV, Coetzee JC. Treatment of primarily ligamentous Lisfranc joint injuries: primary arthrodesis compared with open reduction and internal fixation. A prospective, randomized study. J Bone Joint Surg Am 2006;88(3):514–20.

14. Vertullo CJ, Nunley JA. Participation in sports after arthrodesis of the foot or ankle. Foot Ankle Int 2002;23(7):625–8.

15. Anderson JG, Bohay DR, Henning JA, et al. ORIF vs. Primary arthrodesis of LisFranc injuries: a prospective randomized trial. Presented at the AAOS Annual meeting. San Diego, February 14-18, 2007. Podium presentation.

16. Komenda GA, Myerson MS, Biddinger KR. Results of arthrodesis of the tarsome-tarsal joints after traumatic injury. J Bone Joint Surg Am 1996;78:1665–76.

High-Energy Foot and Ankle Trauma: Principles for Formulating an Individualized Care Plan

Ivan S. Tarkin, MD[a],*, Aaron Sop, DO[b], Hans-Christoph Pape, MD[b]

KEYWORDS

• Foot • Ankle • Trauma • Staged protocols

Management of high-energy foot and ankle trauma requires a well-coordinated care plan to optimize outcomes while avoiding known complications. A spectrum of injuries can occur including fractures, dislocations, or both. The tenuous soft tissue envelope around the foot and ankle is by definition severely traumatized in all cases. Frequently, joints and fractures are contaminated through traumatic lacerations. Compartment syndrome is commonplace.[1]

This article addresses management principles for optimal treatment of severe foot and ankle trauma. However, each injury has a unique "personality" that requires an individualized plan of care based on the fracture/dislocation pattern, soft tissue injury, and host factors. Staged treatment is the preferred management strategy for limb salvage, understanding that respect and care for the compromised soft tissue sleeve is integral for success. Some injuries, however, may be best served with limb-shortening procedures.

INITIAL CARE PLAN

Ultimate success of the severely traumatized lower extremity is often predicated on timely and appropriate care on presentation. Foot and ankle trauma is a common finding in the polytrauma patient. However, there are frequently more urgent injuries that need to be addressed first. Although concomitant head, chest, abdominal, and spine

[a] University of Pittsburgh Medical Center, Department of Orthopaedic Surgery, Division of Orthopaedic Traumatology, 3471 Fifth Avenue, Pittsburgh, PA 15213 412-605-3252, USA
[b] University of Pittsburgh Medical Center, Division of Orthopedic Trauma, 3471 Fifth Avenue, Pittsburgh, PA 15213, USA
* Corresponding author.
E-mail address: tarkinis@upmc.edu (I.S. Tarkin).

Foot Ankle Clin N Am 13 (2008) 705–723
doi:10.1016/j.fcl.2008.08.002
1083-7515/08/$ – see front matter © 2008 Elsevier Inc. All rights reserved.

trauma take priority, the orthopedic surgeon can certainly provide efficient care to the foot and ankle injury to temporize the limb (**Fig. 1**). It is critical to "stop the cycle of injury" and to provide meticulous wound care. Turchin and colleagues[2] and Tran and Thordarson,[3] using validated outcome measures, determined that polytrauma patients with foot and ankle trauma faired significantly worse than multi-injured patients without foot and ankle injury, highlighting the importance of aggressive care protocols in this patient population.

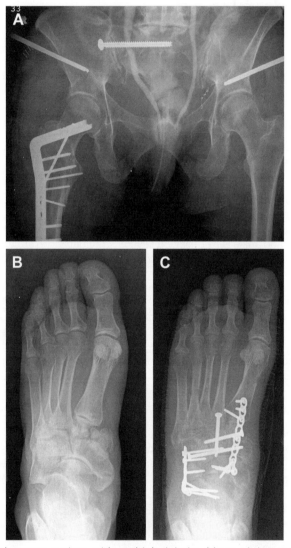

Fig. 1. (*A, B*) Polytrauma patient with multiple injuries (chest, abdomen, pelvis, femur) treated with staged management of bilateral foot and ankle injuries using external fixation on the night of admission. (*C*) Once the patient's medical condition optimized and soft tissue swelling subsided, definitive reconstruction was performed. In the more severe foot, selected fusions were performed including the medial three nonessential midfoot joints as well as the calcaneocuboid joint.

Early care does not mean total care. Typically in the patient with multiple injuries or with isolated musculoskeletal injury, lengthy foot and ankle procedures are not indicated.[4] However, providing basic skeletal stabilization is of critical importance. Fractures and joint dislocations should be adequately reduced. In stable injury patterns splinting will suffice. However, the external fixator is an invaluable tool in more complex skeletal injuries to provide more reliable support.[5]

Open fractures and joints deserve thorough debridement and irrigation to mitigate septic complications infamously reported with these injuries. Furthermore, updating tetanus and antibiotic coverage is the standard of care. Selected uncontaminated Gustillo-Anderson grade I open injuries can be closed primarily after local wound care. However, these traumatic lacerations often should be left open awaiting soft tissue coverage procedures versus delayed primary closure to minimize infectious complications.

INITIAL REDUCTION

Prompt fracture and joint reduction is one of the oldest tenets of orthopedic surgery but must be emphasized in the initial treatment algorithm for the severely traumatized foot and ankle.[6] Improving alignment of the distal extremity is of paramount importance to prevent continued injury to the soft tissue envelope. Widely displaced fractures or major joint dislocations left malpositioned will invariably result in skin compromise or neurovascular embarrassment (**Fig. 2**); unreduced joints are vulnerable to continued irreversible damage to the chondral surfaces leading to posttraumatic arthrosis.

Reduction and splinting in the emergency room after sedation is common practice for most routine foot and ankle fracture/dislocations. However, many high-energy injury patterns are predictably irreducible in this setting and deserve general anesthesia

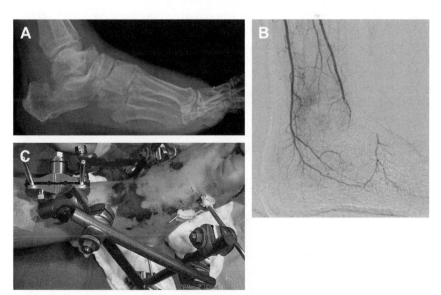

Fig. 2. Complications of untimely reduction. (*A*) Persistently dislocated talus caused full-thickness dorsal skin necrosis and (*B*) disruption of the anterior tibial circulation. (*C*) Chopart dislocation reduced through limited approach to calcaneocuboid joint. Stabilization of calcaneal fracture and Chopart dislocation with external fixation and transarticular K-wires.

with complete muscle relaxation to achieve adequate reduction. Furthermore, unstable patterns typically are best managed in the operating room to perform either temporary or definitive fixation to stabilize fractured anatomy and to maintain joint reductions.

In the initial treatment setting, lengthy reconstructive efforts typically are avoided, especially when the patient presents with multiple injuries after "regular working hours." However, the orthopedic surgeon must be prepared to accomplish the required goals of early care. Mainstays of care include closed manipulation, percutaneous reduction maneuvers, and limited open techniques directed at reducing gross deformity of fractured anatomy and aligning joint dislocations.

STAGED TREATMENT

Definitive reconstruction of high-energy foot and ankle trauma in the acute setting can be fraught with devastating postoperative complications, in that the incidence of wound problems is markedly increased after operation through a swollen, traumatized, soft tissue envelope.[7] Wound breakdown will frequently manifest as either partial- or full-thickness skin necrosis or frank dehiscence of the suture line; these events often are a precursor to deep infection (**Fig. 3**).

In an effort to mitigate these complications, a staged approach often is preferable for managing severe musculoskeletal trauma. This strategy has been particularly successful for decreasing septic complications after pilon fractures (**Fig. 4**).[8,9] Wound problems and deep infections have historically plagued acute reconstruction of the tibial plafond. The principles of staged care can thus be extended to manage other high-energy injuries to the foot and ankle.[10]

In the first stage, gross skeletal deformity is restored and provisionally stabilized. Once the acute soft tissue swelling has resolved, the definitive reconstructive plan is executed to anatomically restore bone and joint injuries.

Benefits of the staged approach are numerous. In the "waiting period" after early care, the surgeon can get to know the patient.[11] Host factors such as age, occupation, recreational activities, and medical comorbidities are analyzed in developing the individualized treatment plan. Interventions are offered in this setting to maximize the patient's overall health status. Nutrition should be optimized. Counseling and treatment are offered to assist with addictions to tobacco, alcohol, and illicit drugs to promote general wellness and improve the success of definitive reconstruction. Realistic expectations and long-term goals are described based on injury severity.

After initial care, the surgeon is afforded an ideal opportunity to develop a precise preoperative plan, which can be executed when systemic and local conditions have improved. Often, adjunctive tests such as computed tomography scans can be

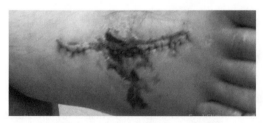

Fig. 3. Acute reconstruction of high-energy Lisfranc fracture dislocation in host with diabetes with resultant partial- and full-thickness skin necrosis, which eventually served as a nidus for deep infection.

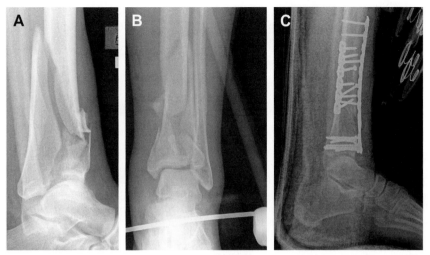

Fig. 4. (*A*) Staged protocol classically described for high-energy pilon fractures. (*B*) A spanning external fixator achieves adequate splinting for the bone and soft tissue injury. (*C*) Definitive reconstruction to obtain anatomic joint restoration proceeds after the soft tissue envelope matures.

ordered to further understand the injury pattern, precisely delineating the bone and joint injuries.[12] Surgical incisions are designed to maximize exposure while minimizing excessive dissection. Reduction strategies are planned and specific implants are ordered to achieve stable accurate foot and ankle reconstruction. The surgeon may realize that referral to a foot and ankle traumatologist is the most prudent course to best serve the patient based on injury complexity.[13]

EXTERNAL FIXATOR AS SKELETAL SPLINT

In the majority of lower energy foot and ankle fractures and dislocations, closed manipulation and splinting is appropriate first-line care. However, with more severe injury patterns, a spanning external fixator is preferable as a temporary "skeletal splint"[14] and must certainly be part of the surgical armamentarium when managing severe foot and ankle trauma.

There are clear advantages and indications for the use of a temporary or definitive external fixator in the management of high-energy foot and ankle trauma. Gross skeletal deformity typically can be reduced by simple distraction alone through Schanz pins strategically placed outside of the zone of injury (**Fig. 5**). Improved bone and joint alignment keeps the soft tissue envelope out to length and helps avoid complications of persistent deformity such as skin and neurovascular embarrassment; patient comfort and mobility are also optimized. Improved skeletal stability and alignment improve local soft tissue conditions to promote early healing. Kinked vascular and lymphatic conduits are re-established, improving local inflow and outflow, promoting resolution of massive swelling and improving local vascularity.

Access to traumatic wounds is facilitated greatly when the external fixator is chosen for early care (**Fig. 6**). Aggressive daily wound care is facilitated by improved access. Consulting services, such as plastic surgeons, can examine the limb to determine need for coverage procedures. Inspection of the overall condition of the distal limb is enhanced to determine timing of further interventions, such as need for

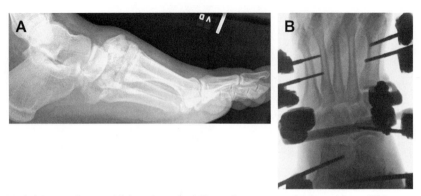

Fig. 5. (*A*) Severe fracture/dislocation of midfoot after motor vehicle accident. (*B*) Improved alignment achieved with both medial and lateral column external fixation. Definitive reconstruction performed 3 weeks from injury.

compartment release or later reconstructive procedures. Furthermore, when repeat interventions in the operating room are required for care of traumatic wounds, the bars and clamps of the external fixator can be removed to deliver care then reassembled.

In most circumstances, the external fixator is used as a temporary device while awaiting soft tissue recovery before precise reduction and definitive internal fixation. However, in selected cases, the fixator stabilizing an adequately reduced severe foot and ankle injury may serve as the preferred treatment.[15,16] Candidates for this treatment are determined based on host and local factors. Patients with substantial medical comorbidities such as peripheral vascular disease or diabetes are at increased risk for wound and septic complications with a more aggressive treatment strategy. Noncompliant patients not possessing the maturity for staged treatment

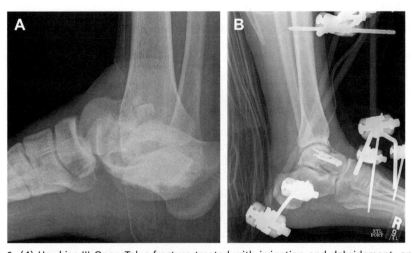

Fig. 6. (*A*) Hawkins III Open Talus fracture treated with irrigation and debridement, open reduction internal fixation, and application of VAC dressing awaiting soft tissue coverage procedure. (*B*) External fixator served two major roles. Intraoperatively, distraction of the hindfoot allowed for reduction of the dislocated talar body. Postoperatively, the fixator stabilized the unstable hindfoot acting as a rigid splint, which allowed access for wound care.

may choose external fixation as a definitive solution. Local conditions of the foot and ankle may furthermore preclude more aggressive open reconstructive efforts.

PERCUTANEOUS TECHNIQUES AND LIMITED OPEN STRATEGIES

In the acute setting, major joint dislocations and gross fracture displacement must be addressed. Although the external fixator is a powerful tool to accomplish this goal, sometimes other methodologies are required. As emphasized, open lengthy surgeries in the initial setting are rarely advisable. However, in most circumstances, percutaneous techniques with or without limited open approaches can accomplish the goals of early care.

Classic examples of cases requiring these techniques include peritalar dislocations[17] and locked Chopart dislocations.[18] Without acute treatment, continued irreversible insult to the neurovascular, cutaneous, and chondral structures continues. Frequently, percutaneous and limited open procedures are necessary for adequate reduction and stabilization.

A specific example is the lateral talus dislocation. The talar head lies medially and is often irreducible with attempted closed reduction, because the talar neck often gets trapped between the posterior tibial tendon and flexor digitorum longus acting as a noose (**Fig. 7**). While dislocated, the medial skin is tented and the posterior medial neurovascular structures are at risk. Prompt open reduction is thus recommended. A strategic transfixion pin can be placed in the calcaneus to gain length on the hindfoot to make room for the talus. Also, Schanz pins can be placed in the talus and first metatarsal base for "joystick" manipulation.

Often, bone and joint reductions are unstable requiring support. Judicious use of temporary K-wire fixation across fractures or joints is prudent in selected cases. Focus must be placed on holding tenuous reductions until typically a more definitive solution can be achieved. If an extended period of K-wire stabilization will be necessary, consideration should be exercised to placing the wires under the skin to mitigate septic complication.

Closure of surgical wounds in this setting may not be advisable. If excessive tension is evident at the time of attempted closure, wounds can be left open. Injudicious tight closures will invariably lead to wound breakdown and septic complications. Delayed primary closure or coverage procedures as necessary can be performed after soft tissue resolution.

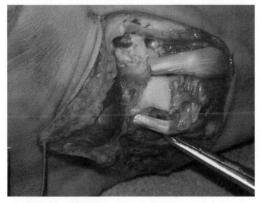

Fig. 7. Irreducible lateral talar dislocation with talar neck trapped between the posterior tibial tendon and flexor digitorum longus.

WOUND MANAGEMENT

A significant percentage of high-energy foot and ankle trauma is accompanied by traumatic laceration. Direct injury to the soft tissues can occur from either blunt or penetrating trauma, but inside-out injuries are common as well. Nonetheless, considering the limited soft tissue sleeve surrounding the foot and ankle, frequently these traumatic wounds communicate with fracture and dislocated joints. Thus, timely, thorough wound care is essential to avoid deep infection.

There is a trend in current clinical practice to primarily close clean uncontaminated lacerations to avoid the necessity for later soft tissue coverage procedures. However, this approach must be used only in circumstances in which a tension-free closure can be performed in a healthy host with an uncontaminated simple wound. All other wounds are best served with serial debridements followed by delayed primary closure or coverage procedure. In other words, when in doubt leave the wound open, perform a second look debridement, and solicit the advice and expertise of a plastic surgery colleague.

INVALUABLE UTILITY OF THE VACUUM-ASSISTED CLOSURE DRESSING

The vacuum-assisted closure (VAC) technique has made a dramatic impact on the care of patients with severe foot and ankle trauma. The VAC assumes many integral roles for promoting healing of both traumatic and surgical wounds after these injuries.

This technique provides negative pressure therapy applied through an open cell-sponge creating an optimized milieu for wound health.[19–21] The VAC removes excessive interstitial fluid, which decreases local edema. This decompresses local vasculature and lymphatics with a resultant increase in microvasculature inflow and lymphatic drainage. The net effect results in improved oxygen tension at the wound site, thereby promoting wound healing and clearance of potential infectious agents. Furthermore, this device promotes the formation of healthy granulation tissue.

The VAC is ideally suited for coverage of traumatic foot and ankle wounds not amenable to primary closure. After leaving the operating room, further contamination of the debrided wound is minimized with the occlusive seal required with this technique. The dressing "prepares" the local wound bed before delayed primary closure or definitive soft tissue coverage.

For smaller wounds, an extended course of VAC treatments can be performed to expedite healing by secondary intention. The dressing is changed every 48 to 72 hours until sufficient granulation tissue response to allow definitive skin grafting. A VAC dressing may also be placed over the skin graft, typically for 5 days, to allow graft maturation and increase graft success rates.

Surgical wounds also benefit from this technique. When foot and ankle incisions are required in the acute setting, primary closure often is not possible or advisable; additionally, incisions created to release compartments are left open (**Fig. 8**). The VAC is used on these wounds until swelling has resolved, and delayed primary closure or coverage is performed.[22]

The VAC can also be applied over surgical wounds closed primarily to replace suction drainage methods. Decreased wound drainage times have been reported.[23] However, this technique demands attention to detail to prevent skin maceration, which can occur if the skin edges are not protected with an occlusive seal.

Finally, in cases of failed primary closure or infected cases, consideration for the VAC is suggested. Debridement must be the first-line treatment. However, a VAC can be used as an adjunctive therapy.[24]

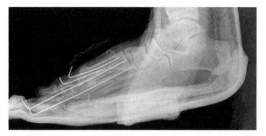

Fig. 8. Compartment syndrome is commonplace with crush injuries to the foot despite simple fracture patterns. Kirshner wire fixation used to stabilize skeletal injury. VAC dressings used to cover/prepare fasciotomy sites before split-thickness skin grafting.

DEFINITIVE RECONSTRUCTION

Once the soft tissue envelope has matured, definitive reconstruction may proceed. In formulating the preoperative plan, a multitude of factors should have influenced decision making including the host and pattern of injury. Bone and joint injuries, as well as the associated soft tissue injuries, have been clearly defined.

Patience is critical when managing these complex foot and ankle injuries. Judgment must be exercised to determine the timing of the definitive surgery, and the answer is often not clearly defined. However, common criteria include the resolution of swelling as evidenced by a "positive wrinkle sign" as well as re-epithelialization of previous fracture blisters (**Fig. 9**).[25] Younger patients with optimal host factors typically can have surgery sooner than those with poorer biologic reserve.

Certainly, extended delays between presentation and definitive operation increase the difficulties associated with achieving anatomic alignment of the bone/joint injuries. The tissues often are "woody," and fractures and joints become more difficult to mobilize.[26] However, the care provided at presentation should have maintained "reasonable" alignment of the skeletal injury up to this point, which therefore highlights the importance of attention to detail at all stages of treatment.

TECHNICAL CONSIDERATIONS

High energy trauma to the foot and ankle typically manifests as multiple fracture/dislocations in a traumatized soft tissue bed. A stepwise approach is always necessary to facilitate a successful surgery. Attention to detail is critical and starts with patient setup.

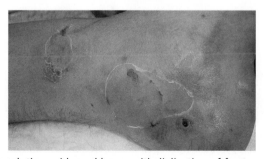

Fig. 9. Soft tissue resolution evidenced by re-epithelialization of fracture blisters.

All surgeries should be performed on a radiolucent operating table with adequate clearance to achieve fluoroscopy without excessive manipulation of the entire leg. Maintaining preliminary reductions can be difficult, and excessive manipulation of the extremity can lead to loss of "perfect" reductions. Frequently, it is advantageous to use "bone foam" to suspend the affected extremity above the contralateral side to facilitate biplanar fluoroscopy and limb access. Also, using an operating table with the ability to "airplane" allows for a comfortable surgical experience when operating on both sides of the foot and ankle. Furthermore, standard equipment should include a headlight to visualize articular reductions.

If a staged procedure was performed with a retained external fixator, the pin sites should be inspected. A fixator often is a useful device to hold fractures and dislocations out to length to facilitate open reduction.[27] Although uncontaminated Schanz pins can be retained, bars and clamps should be removed. Sterile fixator components are used to reassemble the distracter after prepping and draping. Contaminated pins should be removed and pin sites debrided before the open procedure.

RECONSTRUCTIVE PRINCIPLES

It is beyond the scope of this review to discuss in detail all the specific reconstructive techniques necessary to effectively treat high-energy foot and ankle trauma. However, in a large majority of cases, adherence to the basic reconstructive strategies can allow the surgeon the necessary thought processes to design a well-coordinated treatment plan.

In approaching a complex foot and ankle fracture/dislocation, the essential joints should be preserved whenever possible.[28] Anatomic restoration and rigid fixation of intra-articular fractures associated with these joints should be a priority. Instability at the essential joints should be managed with temporary external fixation, trans-articular K-wire fixation, or bridge plating. Nonessential joints can be managed more aggressively with more rigid transarticular fixation after anatomic restoration (**Fig. 10**).

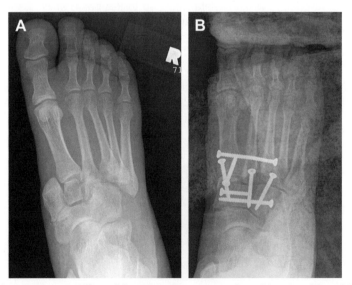

Fig.10. (*A*) High-energy midfoot dislocation after motorcycle accident involving Lisfranc and intercuneiform joints (*B*) treated with open reduction internal fixation using transarticular screws.

SELECTED FUSIONS

Joint preservation is typically the preferred approach when managing foot and ankle trauma, particularly with respect to joints essential to function. For example, in cases of hindfoot fracture/dislocation, intra-articular injuries involving the tibiotalar, subtalar, and talonavicular joints are best served with anatomic reconstruction when possible (**Fig. 11**). However, there is an increasing body of evidence to suggest that selected fusion of nonessential joints is a viable treatment strategy for selected foot fractures/dislocations.[29–31] These techniques often are necessary when treating severely comminuted fracture patterns, particularly in the midfoot.

High-energy midfoot injuries often involve fractures and dislocations at multiple levels. In these instances, a rational treatment plan may consist of bridge plating across the comminuted zones of injury after determining length, alignment, and rotation of the involved column.

When fusion is desired, the remaining joint surfaces are first prepared by removal of the remaining cartilage. The alignment of the column then is achieved by reconstructing major fracture fragments to determine an appropriate "read" on the involved column. Apposition and compression of the remaining joint surfaces often is achieved with compression plating or lag screw fixation when possible.

IMPLANT SELECTIONS

A wealth of implants is currently available to maintain reduction after skeletal reconstruction. Implant selection is based on achieving sufficient stability without excessive bulky hardware. In severe foot and ankle trauma, the primary complications are related to wound problems and deep infection. Lower profile implants are thus preferred. Small and minifragment implants are the most typical devices used in foot

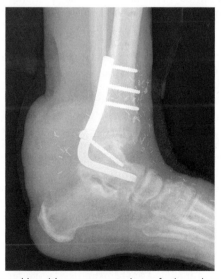

Fig. 11. Grossly unstable ankle with severe posterior soft tissue loss including the Achilles complex and posterior tibiotalar capsule/ligamentous structures. Patient chose limb salvage, although amputation was offered. Care plan consisted of initial external fixation and serial irrigation and debridement awaiting optimization of general health and nutrition in this polytrauma patient. Definitive reconstruction with tibiotalar fusion using posterior blade plate and free flap coverage by plastic surgery service.

and ankle trauma. Specialty precontoured plates are also particularly useful for fractures of the calcaneus, talus, cuboid, and navicular; these implants commonly are engineered with locking technology for use in highly comminuted fractures.

Midfoot fracture/dislocations are managed often with screws alone for nonessential joints placed with or without compression depending on whether arthrodesis is desired. However, often, plating is indicated in the face of comminuted fractures adjacent to midfoot joints.[32,33] Minifragment (2.0, 2.4, or 2.7 mm) plates are most commonly chosen to maximize stability without excessive prominence. In comminuted column injuries, specialty combination plates can be used to enhance fixation with locking technology as well as impart bidirectional compression across joints when arthrodesis is desired.

Kirshner wires (K-wires) should be available to supplement fixation. K-wires are integral as temporary transarticular fixation for unstable essential joints after anatomic joint reconstruction.[34] Also, K-wire fixation can be used in isolation for foot and ankle injuries. However, K-wires alone have an inferior track record as definitive treatment of midfoot fracture/dislocations and should be reserved for cases associated with severely compromised soft tissues or poor host characteristics.[35,36]

Finally, the external fixator is indicated for use after reconstruction to serve as a rigid splint. The fixator supplements the formal reconstruction and soft tissue envelope to encourage uneventful healing and obviates the need for plaster splinting, allowing access to the soft tissue sleeve to facilitate wound care.

LIMB PRESERVATION VERSUS AMPUTATION

Decision making is critical when managing severely traumatized lower extremities. Limb salvage initially is the preferred option by most patients. However, objective reasoning and judgment may suggest that some cases are better served by limb- shortening procedures. Amputation must be considered a viable management strategy rather than a failure of treatment. Results of the LEAP study showed that there was no significant difference in functional outcome between limb salvage and amputation at 7 years.[37] However, acute amputation has been shown to decrease the number of reoperations and rehabilitation time.[38]

A multidisciplinary approach is warranted when determining the best course of action after severe foot and ankle trauma. Essential consultants include a general medicine doctor to identify and potentially modulate host factors such as glucose control in the diabetic and tobacco cessation in the face of addiction. The expertise of a plastic surgeon is typically necessary when local or free flap coverage is required. A vascular surgeon is of obvious benefit in cases of circulatory embarrassment but is also helpful in determining wound healing potential based on perfusion of the traumatized limb. Psychological consultation is used to assess the maturity of the individual choosing limb salvage, which typically requires multiple surgeries, extended hospital stays, significant delays in return to work, and frequent complications.

In most cases, on the day of admission, the patient's injured extremity is "temporized" by performing wound management and open fracture care as well as preliminary alignment procedures such as closed reduction of fractures and external fixation. In the case of a mangled lower extremity, acute amputation is performed on presentation to avoid an emotional attachment to a lower extremity that is beyond reconstruction. This allows the patient and family to positively focus on rehabilitation after wound healing.[39]

In the salvaged limb, more information is collected to formulate a rationale treatment plan. The anticipated plan for reconstruction is described to the patient including potential complications, projected outcome, and rehabilitation time course. The patient's immediate and long-term goals are assessed, which must coincide with the anticipated treatment plan. The patient then decides whether they are dedicated to the process of limb salvage or amputation as a definitive reconstructive procedure.

Objective Studies

Objective data are always helpful for rationale decision making. Factors critical to the success of treatment of the severely traumatized foot and ankle include systemic and local conditions affecting the healing process. Commonly, the patient's nutrition status and lower extremity perfusion are determined to assess healing potential. These factors will influence recommendations for limb salvage versus amputation. Furthermore, if amputation is chosen, these data can influence the type/level of limb shortening procedure performed.

Assessment and optimization of nutritional status is integral in the patient with severe trauma to the foot and ankle. The malnourished patient is at increased risk for wound healing problems, infection, and nonunion after fracture.[40] Routine blood work can establish objective data on nutritional state. A serum albumin level less than 3.5 g/dL or a total lymphocyte count less than 1500 cells/mL is consistent with malnourishment.

Dickhaut and colleagues[41] studied wound healing after Syme amputation, comparing patients' nutritional parameters. Of those with a serum albumin and total lymphocyte count greater than 3.5 g/dL and 1500 cells/mL, 86% healed compared with 18% who were clinically malnourished. A study by Kay and colleagues[42] confirmed the correlation showing that 94% of nourished patients went on to uneventful healing after amputation versus 44% in malnourished patients.

In addition to optimal nutrition, uneventful healing of traumatized musculoskeletal tissues requires adequate local perfusion. Objective tests such toe pressures, transcutaneous oxygen pressures, Doppler ultrasound, or angiography may be helpful if the patient has an ankle brachial index less than 0.9 or nonpalpable pulses. Toe pressures[43] greater than 45 mm Hg and transcutaneous oxygen pressures[44] greater than 30 both correlate with wound healing.

Role of Scoring Systems

Objective scoring systems are available to help determine candidacy for limb salvage versus amputation. However, clinical judgment using a multidisciplinary approach often is more useful for decision making considering the host and specific injury pattern. Of all of the systems, the mangled extremity severity score (MESS) has been shown to be the most useful for calculating which limbs are best served with amputation versus attempts at salvage.[45] However, Bosse and colleagues[46] comprehensively evaluated these scoring systems that attempt to predict amputation versus salvage outcomes and determined that they could not recommend the use of any of them secondary to poor sensitivity.

In the acute setting, the only absolute indication for amputation is irreparable vascular injury in an ischemic limb. A relative indication for amputation is a patient with severe associated systemic injuries. Severe soft tissue loss that would require an extensive reconstructive process that is not compatible with the patient's physiology or request may benefit from amputation. Recently, absence of plantar sensation without documented nerve disruption is no longer considered an absolute indication for amputation.[47]

Amputation Considerations

The goals of lower extremity amputation after trauma are to create a painless, durable, functional limb. Treatment tenants include preservation of residual limb length without compromising soft tissue coverage. Consideration must also be given to muscle balancing of the residual limb and prosthetic wear.

Amputation level is dictated by the extent of bone and soft tissue injury. Preserving length is beneficial, but uneventful healing and comfortable prosthetic fitting typically are more important considerations. Residual limb length is important because the energy required for walking is inversely proportional to the length of the remaining limb.[48] However, achieving more length at the expense of poor stump soft tissue coverage is not advisable. For instance, the use of skin grafting techniques over the distal stump in an effort to preserve length generally should be avoided. Skin grafts typically are not durable enough to withstand the shear forces generated at the skin–prosthesis interface or on the plantar surface of a weight-bearing extremity. Furthermore, fractures above the level of the amputation have worse clinical outcomes, and this should be considered when determining the level of amputation.[49]

Limb-Shortening Procedures

Several concepts must be understood regarding foot amputations. First, a transmetatarsal amputation is the most distal foot amputation that does not require any prosthesis for normal shoe wear (**Fig. 12**).[50] Lisfranc and Chopart amputations historically have had poor outcomes secondary to equinus and equinovarus deformity. However, improvements in surgical technique and prosthetic fitting have made amputation at these levels a viable alternative for severe traumatic foot injuries. At surgery, success is predicated on muscle balancing and heel cord lengthening.[51,52]

The Syme amputation is also an alternative, and it is the most proximal amputation level, allowing the patient to ambulate for short distances without a prosthesis. This amputation is contraindicated in the patient with peripheral vascular disease.[53] Attention to detail is required for this amputation to prevent wound problems and heel pad migration.

Transtibial amputation remains the workhorse level for limb shortening after acute trauma. Most patients undergoing below-the-knee amputation are successful using a prosthesis. Technical considerations include the performance of myocutaneous posterior flap when possible, beveling the anterior tibia at a 30° angle, and performing fibula resection 1 to 2 cm shorter than the tibia in an effort to create a durable painless

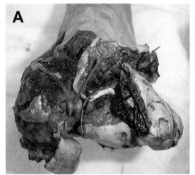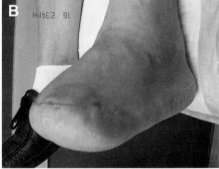

Fig. 12. (*A*) Lawn mower injury treated definitively with transmetatarsal amputation after serial debridements. (*B*) Durable plantar skin used for coverage over distal stump.

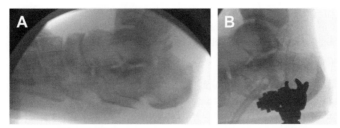

Fig. 13. (*A*) Open calcaneal fracture (primarily extra-articular) treated with serial irrigation and debridement and (*B*) external fixation as definitive treatment in this unhealthy host.

stump.[54] After wound healing, early prosthetic fitting and maximizing knee motion is optimal care.

OUTCOMES

As a group, the majority of high-energy foot and ankle injuries deserve a guarded prognosis.[55] Although these injuries share commonality based on the magnitude of energy imparted to the skeleton and soft tissues, each case has its unique personality. Specific variables influence ultimate outcome including injury pattern, host factors, and treatment. This assessment, however, is based on the limited data available primarily from small retrospective case series.

Severe foot and ankle trauma is often grouped based on the specific skeletal injury pattern. Commonly reported injuries include fracture/dislocation patterns involving the calcaneous, talus, and midfoot. However, the most severe injuries often involve multiple bones and joints in the hindfoot, midfoot, and forefoot.

For example, the literature would suggest that open calcaneal fractures have less than optimal outcomes. However, overall results and complications are typically predicated on the severity and management of the soft tissues injury (**Fig. 13**).[56–59]

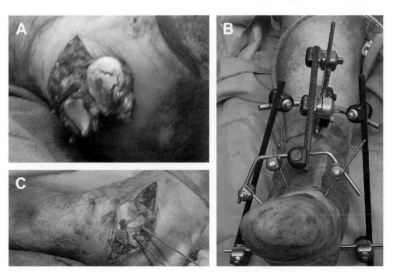

Fig. 14. Talar extrusions. (*A, B*) Pure open peritalar extrusion managed with irrigation and debridement, reduction, and external fixation. (*C*) Body fracture dislocation treated with irrigation and debridement, open reduction internal fixation, and external fixation. Neither patient had septic complication, but both have chronic pain, stiffness, and limp.

A guarded prognosis is particularly evident when considering severe foot and ankle trauma that includes peritalar fracture or dislocation. Open talar neck injuries have the highest risk of complication including a 38% rate of infection.[60] However, other injury patterns such as peritalar dislocations commonly have compromised outcomes (**Fig. 14**).[61,62]

Fracture/dislocation patterns involving the midfoot are commonplace after severe trauma. Variables affecting outcomes are dependent on the degree of initial injury, treatment strategy, and final alignment. Myerson and colleagues[63] determined that the amount of articular damage and the quality of reduction had the greatest impact on final results. Similarly, Arntz and colleagues[64] showed that all Lisfranc injuries in their series that were not anatomically reduced showed moderate to severe posttraumatic arthritis.

SUMMARY

Care of the patient with high-energy foot and ankle trauma requires an individualized care plan. Staged treatment respecting the traumatized soft tissue envelope is often advisable. Wound care is a priority, and the VAC dressing serves an integral role. Before definitive reconstruction, the surgeon needs to develop a treatment plan designed to match the unique personality of the patient and injury. Amputation is considered a rationale treatment option for the patient with severe injury and poor host biology. Despite the most appropriate management, many severe foot and ankle injuries have a guarded prognosis.

REFERENCES

1. Myerson MS. Management of compartment syndromes of the foot. Clin Orthop 1991;271:239–48.
2. Turchin DC, Schemitsch EH, McKee MD, et al. Do foot injuries significantly affect the functional outcome of multiply injured patients? J Orthop Trauma 1999;13(1): 1–4.
3. Tran T, Thordarson D. Functional outcome of multiply injured patients with associated foot injury. Foot Ankle Int 2002;23(4):340–3.
4. Pape HC, Giannoudis PV, Krettek C, et al. Timing of fixation of major fractures in blunt polytrauma: role of conventional indicators in clinical decision making. J Orthop Trauma 2005;19(8):551–62.
5. Rammelt S, Biewener A, Grass R, et al. [Foot injuries in the polytraumatized patient]. Unfallchirurg 2005;108(10):858–65 [In German].
6. Clark WA. History of fracture treatment up to the sixteenth century. J Bone Joint Surg Am 1937;19:47–63.
7. McFerran MA, Smith SW, Boulas HJ, et al. Complications encountered in the treatment of pilon fractures. J Orthop Trauma 1992;6(2):195–200.
8. Sirkin M, Sanders R, DiPasquale T, et al. A staged protocol for soft tissue management in the treatment of complex pilon fractures. J Orthop Trauma 1999;13(2): 78–84.
9. Patterson MJ, Cole JD. Two-staged delayed open reduction and internal fixation of severe pilon fractures. J Orthop Trauma 1999;13(2):85–91.
10. Kuo RS, Tejwani NC, Digiovanni CW, et al. Outcome after open reduction and internal fixation of Lisfranc joint injuries. J Bone Joint Surg Am 2000;82-A(11): 1609–18.
11. Cole PA, Benirschke SK. Minimally invasive surgery for the pilon fracture: the percutaneous-submuscular plating technique. Tech Orthop 1999;14:201–8.

12. Tornetta P 3rd, Gorup J. Axial computed tomography of pilon fractures. Clin Orthop Relat Res 1996;323:273–6.
13. Cutler L, Boot DA. Complex fractures, do we operate on enough to gain and maintain experience? Injury 2005;36(6):804.
14. Tarkin IS, Cole PA. Pilon fracture DiGiovanni and Griesberg core knowledge in orthopedics. Foot and Ankle 2007;252–66.
15. Besch L, Radke B, Mueller M, et al. Dynamic and functional gait analysis of severely displaced intra-articular calcaneus fractures treated with a hinged external fixator or internal stabilization. J Foot Ankle Surg 2008;47(1):19–25.
16. Chandran P, Puttaswamaiah R, Dhillon MS, et al. Management of complex open fracture injuries of the midfoot with external fixation. J Foot Ankle Surg 2006;45(5):308–15.
17. Tucker DJ, Burian G, Boylan JP. Lateral subtalar dislocation: review of the literature and case presentation. J Foot Ankle Surg 1998;37(3):239–47.
18. Klaue K. Chopart fractures. Injury 2004;35(Suppl 2):SB64–70.
19. Morykwas MJ, Argenta LC, Shelton-Brown EI, et al. Vacuum-assisted closure: a new method for wound control and treatment: animal studies and basic foundation. Ann Plast Surg 1997;38(6):553–62.
20. Argenta LC, Morykwas MJ. Vacuum-assisted closure: a new method for wound control and treatment: clinical experience. Ann Plast Surg 1997;38(6):563–76.
21. Buttenschoen K, Fleischmann W, Haupt U, et al. The influence of vacuum assisted closure on inflammatory tissue reactions in the post-operative course of ankle fractures. Foot and Ankle Surg 2007;7:165–73.
22. Tarkin IS, Clare MP, Marcantonio A, et al. An update on the management of high-energy pilon fractures. Injury 2008;39(2):142–54.
23. Stannard JP, Robinson JT, Anderson ER, et al. Negative pressure wound therapy to treat hematomas and surgical incisions following high-energy trauma. J Trauma 2006;60(6):1301–6.
24. Leininger BE, Rasmussen TE, Smith DL, et al. Experience with wound VAC and delayed primary closure of contaminated soft tissue injuries in Iraq. J Trauma 2006;61(5):1207–11.
25. Strauss EJ, Petrucelli G, Bong M, et al. Blisters associated with lower-extremity fracture: results of a prospective treatment protocol. J Orthop Trauma 2006;20(9):618–22.
26. White T, Kennedy S, Cooke C, et al. Primary internal fixation of AO Type C pilon fractures is safe. Orthopaedic Trauma Association Proceedings 2006.
27. Thompson MC, Mormino MA. Injury to the tarsometatarsal joint complex. J Am Acad Orthop Surg 2003;11(4):260–7.
28. Pinney SJ, Sangeorzan BJ. Fractures of the tarsal bones. Orthop Clin North Am 2001;32:21–33.
29. Coetzee JC, Ly TV. Treatment of primarily ligamentous Lisfranc joint injuries: primary arthrodesis compared with open reduction and internal fixation. Surgical technique. J Bone Joint Surg Am 2007;89(Suppl 2 Pt 1):122–7.
30. Mulier T, Reynders P, Dereymaeker G, et al. Severe Lisfrancs injuries: primary arthrodesis or ORIF? Foot Ankle Int 2002;23(10):902–5.
31. Alberta FG, Aronow MS, Barrero M, et al. Ligamentous Lisfranc joint injuries: a biomechanical comparison of dorsal plate and transarticular screw fixation. Foot Ankle Int 2005;26(6):462–73.
32. Schildhauer TA, Nork SE, Sangeorzan BJ. Temporary bridge plating of the medial column in severe midfoot injuries. J Orthop Trauma 2003;17(7):513–20.

33. Cammack PM, Donahue MP, Manoli A 2nd. The bridge and barrel hoop plates as alternatives to external fixation techniques in the foot and ankle. Foot Ankle Clin 2004;9(3):625–36.

34. Wagner R, Blattert TR, Weckbach A. Talar dislocations. Injury 2004;35(Suppl 2): SB36–45.

35. Sangeorzan BJ, Veith RG, Hansen ST Jr. Salvage of Lisfranc's tarsometatarsal joint by arthrodesis. Foot Ankle 1990;10(4):193–200.

36. Lee CA, Birkedal JP, Dickerson EA, et al. Stabilization of Lisfranc joint injuries: a biomechanical study. Foot Ankle Int 2004;25(5):365–70.

37. MacKenzie EJ, Bosse MJ, Kellam JF, et al. Long term persistence of disability following severe lower-limb trauma. J Bone Joint Surg 2005;87A:1801–9.

38. Busse JW, Jacobs CL, Swiontkowski MF, et al. Complex limb salvage or early amputation for severe lower limb injury: a meta-analysis of observational studies. J Orthop Trauma 2007;21(1):70–6.

39. Hansen ST Jr. Salvage or amputation after complex foot and ankle trauma. Orthop Clin North Am 2001;32(1):181–6.

40. Jensen JE, Jensen TG, Smith TK, et al. Nutrition in orthopaedic surgery. J Bone Joint Surg 1982;64A:1263.

41. Dickhaut SC, DeLee JC, Page CP, et al. Nutritional status: importance in predicting wound-healing after amputation. J Bone Joint Surg 1984;66A:71.

42. Kay SP, Moreland JR, Schmitter E, et al. Nutritional status and wound healing in lower extremity amputations. Clin Orthop Relat Res 1987;217:253–6.

43. Pinzur MS, Sage R, Stuck R, et al. Transcutaneous oxygen as a predictor of wound healing in amputations of the foot and ankle. Foot Ankle 1992;13:271.

44. Bone GE, Pomajzl MJ. Toe blood pressure by photoplethysmography: an index of healing in forefoot amputation. Surgery 1981;89(5):569–74.

45. Helfet DL, Howey T, Sanders R, et al. Limb salvage versus amputation. preliminary results of the mangled extremity severity score. Clin Orthop Relat Res 1990;256:80–6.

46. Bosse MJ, MacKenzie EJ, Kellam JF, et al. A prospective evaluation of the clinical utility of the lower-extremity injury severity scores. J Bone Joint Surg 2001; 83A:3–14.

47. Bosse MJ, McCarthy ML, Jones AL, et al. The insensate foot following severe lower extremity trauma: an indication for amputation? J Bone Joint Surg 2005; 87A:2601–8.

48. Waters RL, Perry J, Antonelli D, et al. Energy cost of walking of amputees. The influence of level of amputation. J Bone Joint Surg 1976;58A:42–6.

49. Millstein SG, McCowan SA, Hunter GA, et al. Traumatic partial foot amputations in adults, a long term review. J Bone Joint Surg 1988;70B:251–4.

50. Early JS. Transmetatarsal and midfoot amputations. Clin Orthop Relat Res 1999; 361:85–90.

51. Letts M, Pyper A. The modified Chopart's amputation. Clin Orthop 1990;256: 44–9.

52. Lieberman JR, Jacobs RL, Goldstock L, et al. Chopart amputation with percutaneous heel cord lengthening. Clin Orthop Relat Res 1993;296:86–91.

53. Jany RS, Burkus JK. Long-term follow-up of Syme amputations for peripheral vascular disease associated with diabetes mellitus. Foot Ankle 1988;9(3):107–10.

54. Smith DG, Fergason JR. Transtibial amputations. Clin Orthop Relat Res 1999;361: 108–15.

55. Myerson MS, McGarvey WC, Henderson MR, et al. Morbidity after crush injuries to the foot. J Orthop Trauma 1994;8(4):343–9.

56. Siebert CH, Hansen M, Wolter D, et al. Follow-up evaluation of open intra-articular fractures of the calcaneus. Arch Orthop Trauma Surg 1998;117:442–7.
57. Lawrence SJ, Grau GF. Evaluation and treatment of open calcaneal fractures: a retrospective review. Orthopedics 2003;26:621–6.
58. Berry GK, Stevens DG, Kreder HJ, et al. Open fractures of the calcaneus: a review of treatment and outcome. J Orthop Trauma 2004;18:2002–206.
59. Aldridge JM 3rd, Easley M, Nunley JA, et al. Open calcaneal fractures: results of operative treatment. J Orthop Trauma 2004;18:7–11.
60. Marsh JL, Saltzman CL, Iverson M, et al. Major open injuries of the talus. J Orthop Trauma 1995;9:371–6.
61. Goldner JL, Poletti SC, Gates HS III, et al. Severe open subtalar dislocations. J Bone Joint Surg 1995;77A:1075–9.
62. Merchan EC. Subtalar dislocations: long term follow up of 39 cases. Injury 1992; 23:97–100.
63. Myerson MS, Fisher RT, Burgess AR, et al. Fracture dislocations of the tarsometatarsal joints: end results correlated with pathology and treatment. Foot Ankle 1986;6:225–42.
64. Arntz CT, Veith RG, Hansen ST Jr, et al. Fractures and fracture dislocations of the tarsometatarsal joint. J Bone Joint Surg 1988;70A:173–81.

Distal Tibia Nonunions

Lori K. Reed, MD[a],*, Matthew A. Mormino, MD[a]

KEYWORDS

• Distal • Tibia • Nonunions • Malunions

Distal tibia metaphyseal fractures uncommonly lead to nonunions and malunions. Nonunion rates are reported in the literature to be from 1%–17%.[1,2] McKibbin[3] and Charnley and Baker[4] showed that the healing of periarticular cancellous bone occurs rapidly and it differs from healing of compact or cortical bone in several ways. One of the differences involves creeping substitution; in cancellous bone, the new bone has an existing surface of trabecula to use as a scaffold. Another reason for the paucity of metaphyseal nonunions is the abundant blood supply. A rich network of metaphyseal vessels that anastomose with nutrient arteries supplies sufficient vascularity for fracture healing.[5–7]

Despite the anatomic advantages, metaphyseal nonunions and malunions do occur. Multiple factors can lead to metaphyseal nonunions. Medical comorbidities, tobacco use and poor nutrition are well-known causes of nonunions. Technique-related factors are particularly common to metaphyseal nonunions. Inadequate initial fixation in the metaphyseal segment leads to excess motion at the fracture site, thus leading to fracture nonunion. These nonunions and malunions can cause significant functional disability[8] and they can be particularly challenging to treat. The periarticular metaphyseal fragment is, frequently, small and osteopenic, which makes it difficult to obtain secure fixation. The soft-tissue envelope is commonly tenuous and compromised due to prior surgery.

Treatment options for distal tibial nonunions are limited. The three most common techniques described in the literature are intramedullary nailing, fine wire/ring external fixation, and blade plate reconstruction.

INTRAMEDULLARY NAILING

Intramedullary nailing is the standard operative treatment of diaphyseal tibia fractures[9] It is also used effectively in treatment of nonunions of the tibial shaft.[10–19] Modern nail designs have better distal locking options and the nails can be used in more distal fractures and nonunions.[20] An advantage of intramedullary nailing is that it may be done with less soft tissue disruption than plating, depending on the degree of deformity and the presence of prior instrumentation.[21] Because the nail is a load-sharing

[a] Department of Orthopaedic Surgery and Rehabilitation, University of Nebraska Medical Center, 981080 Nebraska Medical Center, Omaha, NE 68198-1080, USA
* Corresponding author.
E-mail address: lreed@unmc.edu (L.K. Reed).

Foot Ankle Clin N Am 13 (2008) 725–735
doi:10.1016/j.fcl.2008.09.001
1083-7515/08/$ – see front matter © 2008 Elsevier Inc. All rights reserved.

foot.theclinics.com

versus load-bearing device, earlier weight-bearing may be possible. Also, the device is buried, making it a particularly attractive option with a tenuous soft tissue envelope.[21]

McLaren and Blokker[22] treated seven distal tibia nonunions or malunions with locked intramedullary rod fixation. All operative sites healed in an average of 18 weeks. Time to mature bony union and unprotected ambulation was 7.4 months. Complications included shortening, compartment syndrome, residual deformity, loss of ankle motion, and discomfort at the end of the rod requiring removal. Technical difficulties were encountered when the distal fragment was short. This problem was remedied by cutting off the tip of the rod distal to the locking holes. However, McLaren and Blokker believed that this was "stretching the application of this technique."

More recently, Richmond and colleagues,[21] reported on 32 patients with nonunions of the distal fourth of the tibia (**Fig. 1**) which were treated with reamed, locked intramedullary nailing (Synthes USA, Paoli, PA). Twenty-nine of 32 patients were healed in an average of 3.5 months. Two patients united after dynamization and a third patient united 4 months after exchange nailing. Deformity was corrected to a maximum of 4° in all planes.

A femoral distractor was used for deformity correction, with the distractor placed on the concave side if coronal plane deformity was present. (**Fig. 2**) The fracture site was opened in 17 patients if implant removal was required or if the deformity could not be corrected closed. A fibular osteotomy was performed in two patients in whom the deformity still could not be corrected. This was most helpful when translational deformity was present. Reamed intramedullary nailing was performed using a standard medial parapatellar approach. Hand reamers were used to open the medullary canal before passage of the guide wire. All nails were locked distally with a minimum of two locking bolts in the distal fragment. (**Fig. 3**) Proximally, 22 nails were locked dynamically and 10 were locked statically. Dynamic locking was performed to allow impaction at the nonunion site if the nonunions were transverse or short oblique with less that 50% bone loss. (**Fig. 4**) The intramedullary reamings were used for local bone grafting. In open cases, the reamings were collected and packed into the nonunion site. Cultures were taken directly from the nonunion site in all open nailings and reamings were cultured in closed nailings. All patients were maintained on parenteral antibiotics for 48 hours postoperatively. If intraoperative cultures were positive, patients were placed on directed antibiotic therapy. All patients were allowed to toe-touch weight-bear until

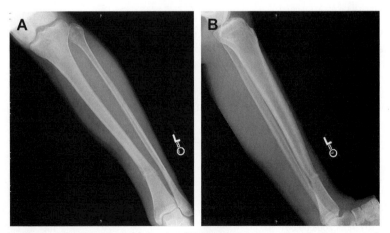

Fig. 1. (*A, B*) Preoperative AP and lateral radiographs distal one-fourth tibia nonunion.

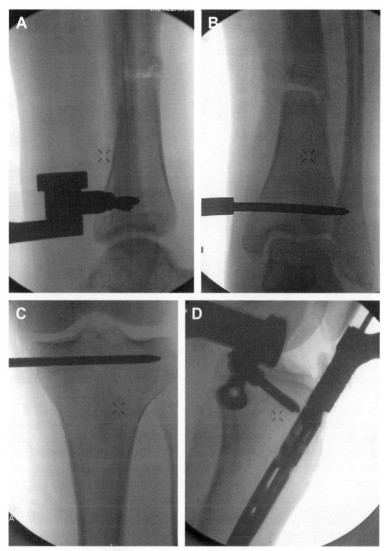

Fig. 2. (*A, B, C, D*) Placement of femoral distractor to correct coronal deformity.

wounds were healed. After the wounds were healed, patients with dynamically locked nails were allowed to weight-bear as tolerated, and patients with statically locked nails were allowed to progress their weight bearing after 6 weeks.

Of particular concern with this technique is its use in tibial nonunions with a history of external fixation or infection. (**Fig. 5**) Several studies,[23–25] however, have demonstrated that this technique may be safe, even if pin tract infection had occurred, as long as there is no drainage at the time of the nailing procedure and the patients are managed aggressively with appropriate antibiotics. Johnson and colleagues,[24] reported on 13 patients with 16 tibia fractures who were initially treated with external fixation and who secondarily had delayed intramedullary nailing after fixator removal. Intramedullary nailing was performed at an average of 13 days after fixator removal.

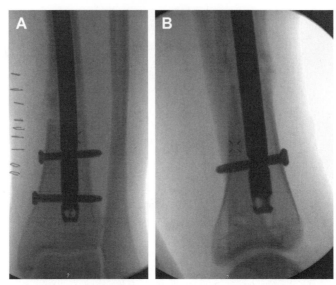

Fig. 3. (A, B) Intraoperative fluoroscopy images of intramedullary nail placement with 3 interlocking screws distal to the fracture site.

Antibiotics were given both preoperatively and postoperatively. All patients healed without evidence of infection at an average of 22.5 months follow-up. Marshall and colleagues[25] reviewed 24 patients in 25 cases who underwent delayed intramedullary (IM) nailing after external fixation. All 25 cases had clinical evidence of pin tract infection before the removal of the external fixator. Intramedullary nailing was not performed until after the pin sites had dried. Only one case resulted in evidence of deep infection being reactivated following IM nailing. The authors concluded that pin tract infection does not seem to be a contraindication to the subsequent use of an IM nail, provided that underlying active osteomyelitis is not present. A delay of 7 to 14 days after removal of the fixator was recommended (**Fig. 6**).

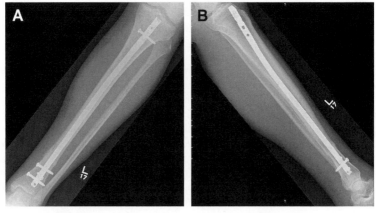

Fig. 4. (A, B) Postoperative radiographs healed nonunion at 3 months.

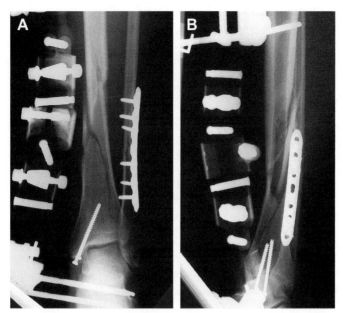

Fig. 5. (*A, B*) Preoperative radiographs of a distal tibia nonunion initially treated with a unilateral external fixator.

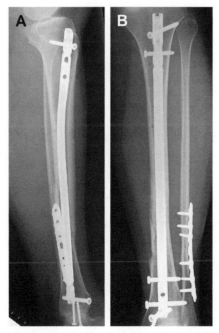

Fig. 6. (*A, B*) The external fixator was removed and the pin sites allowed to seal. Patient was then treated with an intramedullary nail and went on to union without evidence of infection.

Intramedullary nailing for distal tibia nonunions is an attractive option that has been shown to be effective in nonunions with a distal segment large enough to accommodate two distal interlocking screws. However, when the metaphyseal nonunion is more distal and does not allow for adequate interlocking, other treatment modalities must be used.

FINE WIRE/RING EXTERNAL FIXATION

External fixation with a ring fixator can be a useful technique to treat metaphyseal nonunions because it allows for simultaneous correction of deformity, compression of the nonunion, and transport of bone and soft tissues to close defects. Good results have been reported in terms of eventual union and correction of deformity.[26–30]

Lonner and colleagues[31] reviewed 10 nonunions of the distal tibia metaphysis treated with an Ilizarov external fixator. Six patients had a history of osteomyelitis. Bifocal compression–distraction lengthening osteosynthesis was performed in all cases. Ankle arthrodesis was performed in two patients. Eight nonunions healed. Limb length was corrected in five cases; angular and rotational alignment was corrected to within 5 degrees in seven patients. Results were considered good to excellent in seven cases and poor in three. The authors reported a high complication rate, primarily due to pin tract infections. Yet, despite this, they concluded that this technique provides an alternative method for the treatment of difficult problems associated with complex low distal tibial metaphyseal nonunions.

Kabata and colleagues[32] reported seven metaphyseal nonunions with bone loss that were treated with external fixation and distraction osteogenesis. Two of the seven nonunions involved the distal tibia. Five were septic nonunions and two were aseptic. Both distal tibia nonunions were infected. All nonunions healed with no recurrence of infection. The mean external fixation period was 219 days. All patients reported excellent pain reduction. The functional results were classified as excellent in two patients, good in three, and fair in two.

Despite successful treatment of these complicated nonunions, there are disadvantages to this treatment option. There is a significant risk of complications, particularly from pin tract infections. Often times, patients do not tolerate the fixation apparatus well and there is an extended length of time required to achieve union. The use of circular external fixation requires significant technical experience and knowledge of the Ilizarov philosophy.

Sanders and colleagues[33] set out to determine the sources and magnitude of residual morbidity after successful treatment of tibial nonunion using the Ilizarov device and techniques. Residual pain was present in over 90% of patients at a mean follow-up of 39 months. Of these patients, 80% reported the worst pain was in the ankle; less than 10% felt the worst pain in the knee or at the fracture site. Ankle pain with disability was thus determined to be the major source of residual disability.

Although this technique can be successful, its main indication is for infected nonunions with significant bone or soft tissue loss.[34]

BLADE PLATE RECONSTRUCTION

Blade plate fixation offers several advantages when treating these difficult nonunions. The blade has a broad surface to help achieve stable fixation in the small, osteopenic distal segment. It provides a fixed angle that can aid in deformity correction and achieving compression across the nonunion site. It offers fixation that is stable enough to allow early ankle motion, which is one of the primary functional limitations of these patients. This technique has been shown to predictably achieve union with low complication rates as well as improvement in the function of patients treated in this manner.[35–37]

Harvey and colleagues[36] treated 37 periarticular nonunions in 33 patients with locking custom-contoured blade plates. The blade plates were fashioned from standard compression plates: 3.5 mm DCP or LCDCP and 4.5 mm DCP or LCDCP (Synthes, Pennsylvania, USA). Of the nonunions, 13 were implanted in distal tibiae; 17 in proximal tibiae; and three in proximal humeri. Twenty-nine operative sites were treated successfully. Five patients had persistent nonunion, of which four united after a second, custom-contoured blade plate procedure. Sixteen blade plates were performed in patients with a diagnosis of clinical infection and all progressed to union and resolution of infection. Twelve of the 13 implanted in the distal tibia went on to union. Seven patients were treated with free tissue transfers for infection and/or inadequate soft tissue coverage. Patients with a history of osteomyelitis were treated in a staged fashion. They underwent debridement and insertion of antibiotic beads followed at 6 weeks by bead removal, blade plate insertion and/or tissue transfer and/or bone grafting.

Chin and colleagues[37] salvaged 13 distal tibia metaphyseal nonunions with a 90° cannulated blade plate (Synthes, Paoli, PA). Three arthritic tibiotalar joints underwent simultaneous fusion. All 13 patients achieved radiographic and clinic union at an average of 15.6 weeks. Twelve patients had a good clinical result and one patient had a fair result.

The authors of this article[8] reported the functional outcome of 11 patients prospectively followed before and after blade plate reconstruction of distal tibia metaphyseal nonunions. The average duration of the nonunion was 11 months. Patients had undergone an average of 3.1 procedures before blade plate. Three patients had prior deep infections, and one patient had an active infection. A precontoured 4.5 mm cannulated humeral blade plate (Synthes USA, Paoli, PA) (**Fig. 7**) was applied

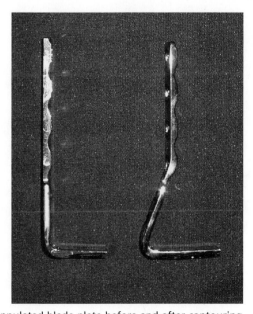

Fig. 7. 90-degree cannulated blade plate before and after contouring.

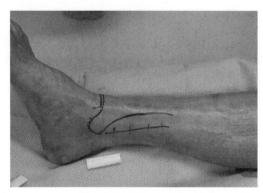

Fig. 8. Posteromedial approach to the distal tibia 1 cm posterior to the medial crest of the tibia.

medially. All patients healed their nonunions, with an average of 16 weeks. The average time to full weight-bearing was 12 weeks. Alignment was improved to an average coronal alignment of 4° of varus and a sagittal alignment of 2° apex posterior angulation. American Orthopaedic Foot and Ankle Society scores improved from an average preoperative score of 29 to an average postoperative score of 89. The lone complication was one deep infection, which was successfully treated with one irrigation and debridement and 6 weeks of parenteral antibiotics.

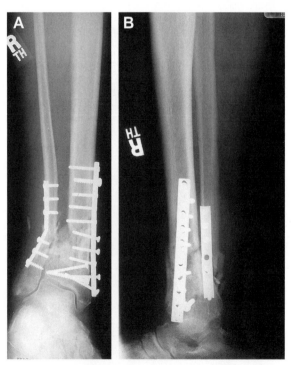

Fig. 9. (*A, B*) Preoperative radiographs of a 5-month old distal tibia nonunion initially treated with standard compression plating.

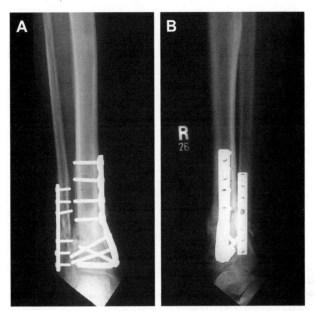

Fig. 10. (*A, B*) Postoperative radiographs at 6 months with healed fracture.

The nonunion was approached through an incision 1 cm posterior to the medial crest of the tibia. (**Fig. 8**) Realignment was accomplished by an osteotomy of the tibial nonunion and facilitated by a fibular osteotomy at approximately the same level. The plate was precontoured from tracings and a bone model was then fixed directly to the medial surface of the tibia. The nonunion sites were not formally taken down or extensively debrided except to contour the bone to allow seating of the plate or to accomplish realignment (**Figs. 9** and **10**). Iliac crest bone graft (eight patients) or local bone graft (three patients) were used to fill bone defects. In the two earliest patients, the fibular osteotomies were plated; in the remaining nine patients, the fibula was not plated. One patient with an active infection required three debridements before fixation and a free flap at the time of fixation. No other patient had wound coverage difficulties despite scarring from prior surgeries.

SUMMARY

Although distal tibia metaphyseal nonunions are uncommon, they do occur and they cause significant functional disability. They remain a challenging therapeutic problem with relatively few treatment options. Circular external fixation is most useful in infected nonunions with significant bone or soft tissue loss.

If the distal segment is large enough, then reamed, locked intramedullary nailing is a good option. If the distal segment it too small to allow for this technique, blade plate reconstruction leads to predictably high healing rates with low complication rates and it remains these authors' treatment of choice.

REFERENCES

1. Ruedi TP, Allgower M. The operative treatment of intra-articular fractures of the lower end of the tibia. Clin Orthop 1979;138:105–10.

2. Teeny SM, Wiss DA. Open reduction and internal fixation of tibial plafond fractures. Clin Orthop 1993;292:108–17.

3. McKibbin B. The biology of fracture healing in long bones. J Bone Joint Surg Br 1978;60:150–62.

4. Charnley J, Baker SL. Compression arthrodesis of the knee: a clinical and histologic study. J Bone Joint Surg Br 1952;34:187–99.

5. Rhinelander FW. Tibial blood supply in relation to fracture healing. Clin Orthop 1974;105:34–81.

6. Rhinelander FW, Baragry RA. Microangiography in bone healing: I. Undisplaced closed fractures. J Bone Joint Surg Am 1962;44:1273–98.

7. Rhinelander FW, Phillips RS, Steel WC, et al. Microangiography in bone healing: II. Displaced closed fractures. J Bone Joint Surg Am 1968;50:643–62.

8. Reed LR, Mormino MA. Functional outcome after blade plate reconstruction of distal tibia metaphyeal nonunions. J Orthop Trauma 2004;18:81–6.

9. Bone LB, Johnson KD. Treatment of tibial fractures by reaming and intramedullary nailing. J Bone Joint Surg Am 1968;68:877–87.

10. Dogra AS, Ruiz AL, Thompson NS, et al. Dia-metaphyseal distal tibia fractures—treatment with a shortened intramedullary nail: a review of 15 cases. Injury 2000; 31:799–804.

11. Bohler J. Treatment of nonunion of the tibia with closed and semiclosed intramedullary nailing. Clin Orthop 1965;43:93–101.

12. Clancey GJ, Winquist RA, Hansen ST. Nonunion of the tibia treated with Kuntscher intramedullary nailing. Clin Orthop 1982;167:191–6.

13. Court-Brown CM, Keating JF, McQueen MM. Exchange intramedullary nailing: its used in aseptic tibial nonunion. J Bone Joint Surg Br 1995;77:407–11.

14. Lottes JO. Treatment of delayed or nonunion fractures of the tibia by a medullary nail. Clin Orthop 1965;43:111–28.

15. Mayo KA, Benirschke SK. Treatment of tibial malunions and nonunions with reamed intramedullary nails. Orthop Clin North Am 1990;21:715–24.

16. Miller ME, Ada JR, Webb LX. Treatment of infected nonunion and delayed union of tibia fractures with locking intramedullary nails. Clin Orthop 1989;245:233–8.

17. Moed BR, Watson JT. Intramedullary nailing of aseptic tibial nonunions without the use of the fracture table. J Orthop Trauma 1995;9:128–34.

18. Templeman D, Thomas M, Varecka T, et al. Exchange reamed intramedullary nailing for delayed union and nonunion of the tibia. Clin Orthop 1995;315:169–75.

19. Wiss DA, Stetson WB. Nonunion of the tibia treated with a reamed intramedullary nail. J Orthop Trauma 1994;8:189–94.

20. Gorczyca JT, McKale J, Pugh K, et al. Modified tibial nails for treating distal tibia fractures. J Orthop Trauma 2002;16:18–22.

21. Richmond J, Colleran K, Borens O, et al. Nonunion of the distal tibia treated by reamed intramedullary nailing. J Orthop Trauma 2004;18:603–10.

22. McLaren AC, Blokker CP. Locked intramedullary fixation for metaphyseal malunion and nonunion. Clin Orthop 1991;265:253–60.

23. Mosheiff R, Safran O, Segal D, et al. The unreamed tibial nail in the treatment of distal metaphyseal fractures. Injury 1999;30:83–90.

24. Johnson EE, Simpson LA, Helfet DL. Delayed intramedullary nailing after failed external fixation of the tibia. Clin Orthop 1990;253:251–7.

25. Marshall PD, Saleh M, Douglas DL. Risk of deep infection with intramedullary nailing following the use of external fixators. J R Coll Surg Edinb 1991;36:268–71.

26. Ebraheim NA, Skie MC, Jackson WT. The treatment of tibial nonunion with angular deformity using an Ilizarov device. J Trauma 1995;38:111–7.

27. Morandi M, Zembo MM, Ciotti M. Infected tibial pseudoarthrosis: a 2-year follow up on patients treated by Ilizarov technique. Orthopedics 1989;12:497–508.
28. Paley D, Chaudray M, Pirone AM, et al. Treatment of malunions and mal-nonunions of the femur and tibia by detailed preoperative planning and the Ilizarov techniques. Orthop Clin North Am 1990;21:667–91.
29. Pearson RL, Perry CR. The Ilizarov technique in the treatment of infected tibial nonunions. Orthop Rev 1989;18:609–13.
30. Schwartsman V, Choi SH, Schwartsman R. Tibial nonunions. Treatment tactics with the Ilizarov method. Orthop Clin North Am 1990;21:639–53.
31. Lonner JH, Koval KJ, Golyakhovsky V, et al. Posttraumatic nonunion of the distal tibial metaphysic. Treatment using the Ilizariv circular external fixator. Am J Orthop 1995 May;(Suppl):16–21.
32. Kabata T, Tsuchiya H, Sakurakichi K, et al. Reconstruction with distraction osteogenesis for juxta-articular nonunions with bone loss. J Trauma 2005;58:1213–22.
33. Sanders DW, Galpin RD, Hosseini M, et al. Morbidity resulting from the treatment of tibial nonunion with the Ilizarov frame. Can J Surg 2002;45:196–200.
34. Ring D, Jupiter JB, Gans BS, et al. Infected nonunion of the tibia. Clin Orthop 1999;369:302–11.
35. Carpenter CA, Jupiter JB. Blade plate reconstruction of metaphyseal nonunion of the tibia. Clin Orthop 1996;332:23–8.
36. Harvey EJ, Henley MB, Swointkowski MF, et al. The use of a locking custom contoured blade plate for peri-articular nonunions. Injury 2003;34:111–6.
37. Chin KR, Nagarkatti DG, Miranda MA, et al. Salvage of distal tibia metaphyseal nonunions with the 9° cannulated blade plate. Clin Orthop 2003;409:241–9.

Surgical Techniques for the Reconstruction of Malunited Ankle Fractures

Anthony Perera, MBChB FRCS(Orth)*, Mark Myerson, MD

KEYWORDS

- Ankle fracture • Ankle malunion • Ankle reconstruction
- Complications

Ankle fractures are so common that there is a certain amount of disregard for the potential for adverse consequences, as most of these injuries do very well.[1] There is clearly an association between malunion of an ankle fracture and poor outcomes requiring some type of reconstruction, and although the latter can be accomplished, it can be very difficult. The key lies in accurate assessment, careful preoperative planning, and then the use of specialized reconstructive techniques. We will describe this process using clinical cases to illustrate the management of malunion.

DIAGNOSIS

It is difficult to accurately assess the direction and magnitude of a malunion, which can occasionally make it difficult to even diagnose. However, the radiological guidelines listed in **Table 1** are useful.

MANAGEMENT

Anatomic reduction after fracture can result in good outcomes and this may be a more important factor than either age or fracture type.[2] Lateral talar shift of more than 1 mm may be sufficient to cause abnormal load bearing of the ankle but realignment of the malunion can reverse this abnormal contact.[3] Thus, secondary reconstruction should always be considered before salvage procedures such as arthrodesis or joint replacement.[4] It is difficult to determine exactly when reconstruction can still be performed, but as a general rule, if malalignment is present and arthritis is not severe, then reconstruction can definitely improve function. Some authors have stated that this

Institute for Foot and Ankle Reconstruction at Mercy, Mercy Medical Center, 301 St. Paul Street, Baltimore, MD 21202, USA
* Corresponding author.
E-mail address: anthony_perera@hotmail.com (A. Perera).

Foot Ankle Clin N Am 13 (2008) 737–751
doi:10.1016/j.fcl.2008.09.005
1083-7515/08/$ – see front matter © 2008 Elsevier Inc. All rights reserved.

foot.theclinics.com

Table 1 Radiographic markers of ankle malunion	
	Consider Reconstruction if:
Medial malunion/Instability	
Medial clear space[17,18]	>4 mm, or > superior space
Talar tilt[18]	>5°
Syndesmosis	
Fibula overlap[18]	<10 mm
Tibiofibular clear space[18]	<5 mm
Talar shift[10]	>1 mm
External rotation stress test[19]	Compare with opposite side
CT scan of syndesmosis[20]	Incongruency
Fibula length	
Talocrural angle[21]	Average = 83° ± 4° but compare with opposite side
Fibula shortening[22]	>2 mm
Fibula rotation	
CT fibula torsional angle[23]	>15°
Distal tibial malunion	
Tibial plafond angle[15]	>10°

reconstruction can be performed up to 1 year after suboptimal fixation.[5] Others, including Kelikian[6] and Marti and Nolte,[7] recommend that it can be considered up to 7 years after injury even when there are degenerative changes, but there is very little evidence-based guidance on this. This notion may well be correct, but as stated it is difficult to give a definite guideline as to timing of this surgery. It would seem obvious that the earlier this intervention is performed, the better, but reconstruction and realignment may be necessary as a staged procedure, even knowing that an arthrodesis or joint replacement is likely in the future (**Figs. 1–3**).

Each individual injury needs to be evaluated on its own merits taking into consideration the function and expectations of the patient, the radiographic measures noted earlier, and the presence and severity of any degenerative changes. The aim of this article is to present the technical aspects of secondary reconstruction and these will be illustrated using clinical examples. The first step is to accurately define the deformity. The radiograph in **Fig. 4** shows a nonunion of the fibula with shortening, external rotation, and valgus deformity. There is a lateral shift of the talus and the valgus talus has resulted in erosion of the lateral tibial plafond. There is widening of the medial gutter and malunion of the medial malleolus. If this each of these issues can be addressed, then this ankle is potentially salvageable (**Figs. 4** and **5**).

Fibula Malunion: Fibula Lengthening and Internal Rotation

The most common scenario of malunion involves shortening and external rotation of the fibula, and reconstruction can yield successful results many years following injury.[8] If there is concurrent opening of the medial joint space it may be necessary to open the medial gutter to clear the fibrous scar tissue that frequently prevents anatomic reduction. It must be performed before attempting the fibula correction because it is difficult to translate the talus if this scar is present, no matter how minor this medial widening appears. This medial gutter debridement can be performed arthroscopically or via an

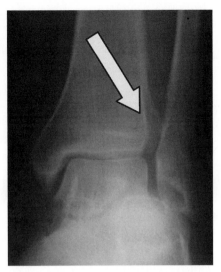

Fig. 1. Tibiofibular clear space.

open arthrotomy, but even with arthrotomy it is difficult to identify the articular surfaces. It is best to begin with sharp dissection with a scalpel. This can then be completed with a fine rongeur to remove the tissue until the cartilage is exposed and reduction of the talus is possible.

1. It can be difficult to judge the required amount of lengthening of the fibula necessary, and comparison radiographs of the contralateral ankle are invaluable in determining the correct length. Intraoperatively the articular contact between the fibula and the lateral edge of the talus can also be directly examined. It is not as easy to determine the rotational correction required. Although a malunited fibula is

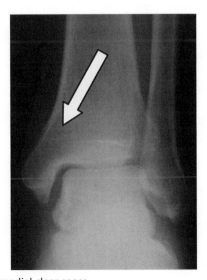

Fig. 2. Widening of the medial clear space.

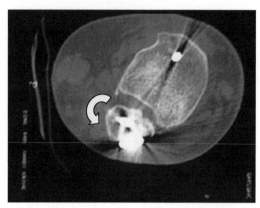

Fig. 3. Displacement and external rotation of the fibular.

generally associated with some external rotation deformity, at times shortening may be the only deformity. Nonetheless, a CT scan is very helpful to determine any rotational deformity that will be necessary.

2. Should the osteotomy be performed at the level of the malunion, or more distally in metaphyseal bone? If external rotation is present, should the osteotomy be performed transversely, or obliquely through the original plane of the fracture? Generally, we find it easier to perform a transverse rather than an oblique osteotomy, leaving sufficient length of the fibula distally for fixation. A transverse osteotomy is made above the level of the syndesmosis allowing sufficient length for distal fixation. An oblique osteotomy can be made through the plane of the original fracture, which will enable correction of length and rotation. While this may be more stable and have better healing potential, it is technically more difficult, and is more difficult to "fine-tune" (**Fig. 6**A).

3. Once the osteotomy has been performed, it is important to shift the distal fibula only, and not allow proximal migration. The proximal fibula is therefore temporarily

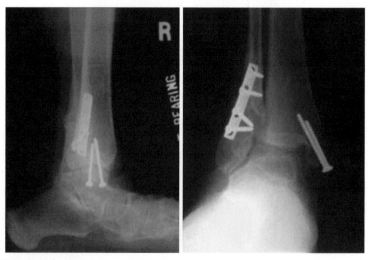

Fig. 4. Malunited fracture.

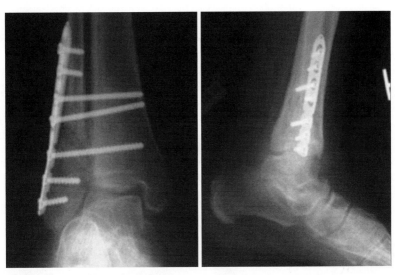

Fig. 5. Ankle after reconstruction.

stabilized with two K-wires into the tibia, so that the distal end moves relative to the stabilized fragment (**Fig. 6**B).

4. The syndesmosis needs to be opened and taken down so that the lateral malleolus can be distracted distally using a lamina spreader while at the same time internally rotated using a bone reduction clamp. It is then transfixed to the tibia using two further K-wires (**Fig. 6**C).
5. A structural allograft is used and inserted into the osteotomy while the distal segment remains distracted (**Fig. 6**D).
6. It is secured using plate fixation, the more distal the osteotomy, the more difficult the fixation, and at times a custom plate may be required. In this particular case, a locking compression plate (Orthohelix, Akron, OH) was used with one screw for stabilization of the syndesmosis. In very osteopenic bone the hold can be improved by using multiple tibial pro-fibular screws. Consideration should be given to fusing the syndesmosis if the deformity is severe or the bone quality poor, but even in these cases a fusion is not necessary if stable fixation can be obtained (**Fig. 6**E–I).[9]

The Syndesmosis

It is generally perceived that widening of the syndesmosis should be reduced and fixed, however there are some unanswered questions. The work by Ramsey and Hamilton[10] (subsequently confirmed by Harper and others)[11] has shown the loading changes that occur with talar shift. What we are not certain of, however, are the long-term consequences of these changes. The decision is straightforward if there is obvious talar tilting and medial opening, but the treatment is not clear if there is an asymptomatic widening of the syndesmosis. There are other situations when it would appear that the syndesmosis may be the source of pain, despite fairly innocuous-looking radiographs. Infiltration of a local anesthetic into the syndesmosis can be useful in diagnosing the source of pain before making clinical decision making. Other issues are how late a delayed reduction can be performed and when would fusion of the syndesmosis be preferable to open reduction and internal fixation? This last dilemma may be a moot point, however, because the procedure of opening the

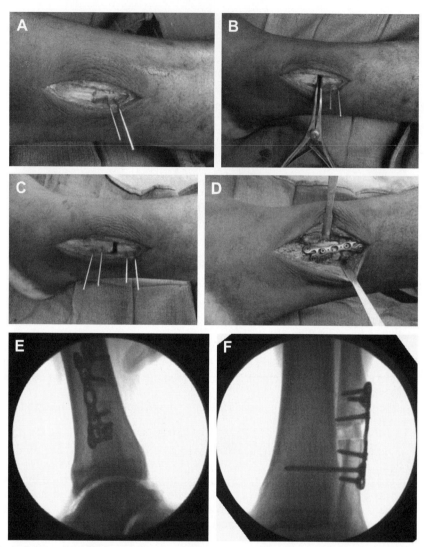

Fig. 6. (A) Proximal fibula stabilization. (B) Distraction of the fibula osteotomy. (C) Stabilization of the distal fibula. (D) Insertion of graft and fixation. (E, F) Intraoperative fluoroscopy post-fixation. (G) Left ankle preoperative. (H) Six-week postoperative AP. (I) Six-week postoperative lateral.

syndesmosis, clearing all the fibrous tissue, and fixing it as described above most likely results in a functional fusion because of the scarring. This can be performed instead of a fusion even after a long delay. Clearly if the instability recurs despite this, then fusion may be the next step.

Deformity of the Tibial Plafond: the use of Tibial Osteotomy and Plafondplasty

The commonest situation in which a plafondplasty may be used is in a valgus malunion of the ankle associated with osteopenia. A nonunion of a fibula fracture or a stress fracture of the fibula associated with severe flatfoot deformity is a typical cause of

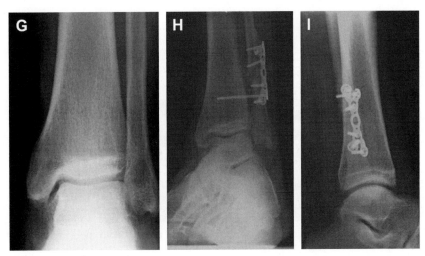

Fig. 6. (*continued*)

this problem (**Fig. 7**). As the ankle drifts into valgus, the talus can impact upon the tibia causing it to collapse laterally. Less commonly it may be seen in a neuropathic ankle with an acute fracture, if it is picked up before it develops into a Charcot joint.

Reconstruction should be considered for any fibula fracture with shortening and valgus malunion. The presence of advanced degenerative change is a relative contra-indication only, because some patients will benefit from reconstruction even in the presence of marked degeneration.[7] This is complicated by the fact that there is no reliable method of qualitatively and quantitatively assessing the degenerative changes. This is especially true in the rheumatoid foot and ankle; these patients toler-ate ankle arthritis fairly well, although hindfoot deformity, particularly valgus, can be quite troublesome.

Surgical planning for correction of a malunion of the fibula with valgus deformity of the plafond requires consideration of the foot as a whole, since the ankle valgus de-formity cannot be corrected on its own. Furthermore, a fixed hindfoot valgus deformity can develop in a patient without a preexisting flatfoot as a result of the combination of ankle valgus and an unstable first ray, and in addition to the tibial correction, a calca-neal osteotomy or arthrodesis of the first tarsometatarsal joint may need to be consid-ered (**Fig. 8A**).

Lateral tibial osteotomy or "plafondplasty" frequently requires both a medial and lateral approach, since scar is frequently present in the medial gutter as noted above. Although it may appear that the deltoid ligament is ruptured, it rarely requires recon-struction, and once the deformity is corrected, medial instability is not common. The lateral incision depends on the level of the fracture but requires an extensile approach as far distally as the sinus tarsi if a hindfoot arthrodesis is performed simul-taneously. Care must be taken if the hindfoot valgus has been present for a long time; if the deformity is fixed there may be problems with closure of a lateral skin incision. It is usually easiest to do the tibial reconstruction first, particularly in very distal fractures of the fibula, as reflection of the fibula in this case requires release of the syndesmotic ligaments necessitating fusion of the syndesmosis (**Fig. 8B**). If the fibula fracture is near the site of the osteotomy it is much easier to perform the reconstruction.

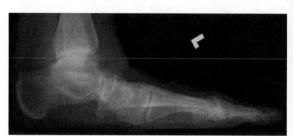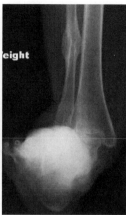

Fig. 7. Malunited stress fracture of the fibula in a patient with preexisting flatfoot deformity.

The tibial plafond is usually compressed anterolaterally; however, it is only possible to perform a uniplanar correction. The osteotomy is planned in such a way that it begins 1 to 2 cm above the plafond with the apex at the most medial extent of the intra-articular deformity. It is important that the osteotomy remains extra-articular ending in the subchondral bone about 5 mm above the joint surface (**Fig. 8**C). This is best planned using a K-wire; the osteotomy is then performed along the wire using a long narrow saw blade under fluoroscopic guidance. The correction is performed very gradually by passing a broad osteotome down and using the viscoelastic properties of the bone to open the osteotomy. A nontoothed laminar spreader can be helpful but should be used in small increments and under image guidance. Once the alignment is corrected, the osteotomy is filled with cancellous bone graft, which heals well in this location. Fixation can be an issue, as a plate can get in the way of fibula reduction, although this can be obviated with the use of a small one third tubular plate placed anteriorly and screws laterally. Generally, however, the osteotomy can be fixed with two or three transverse screws, and the steeper the osteotomy, the easier it is to fix (**Fig. 8**D–F).

The final step is to lengthen and de-rotate the fibula as discussed previously. Occasionally when the fibula is very short it is difficult to know how much correction is required and therefore it may better to get it out to length first, although this can make the tibial osteotomy more difficult.

Varus malunion is much less frequent than valgus deformity; fortunately the surgical planning and technique is more straightforward. The procedure is similar to that used for approaching and grafting osteochondral defects. The osteotomy itself is performed in the same manner as described previously; screw fixation is usually all that is required (**Fig. 9**A).

Medial Malleolus

Malunion of the medial malleolus can lead to a varus or valgus deformity, which is intra-articular, and can be treated either with a simple resection of the prominent impinging bone or by realignment osteotomy. If there is a nonunion, then the correction is straightforward, otherwise the correction may need to made through an oblique

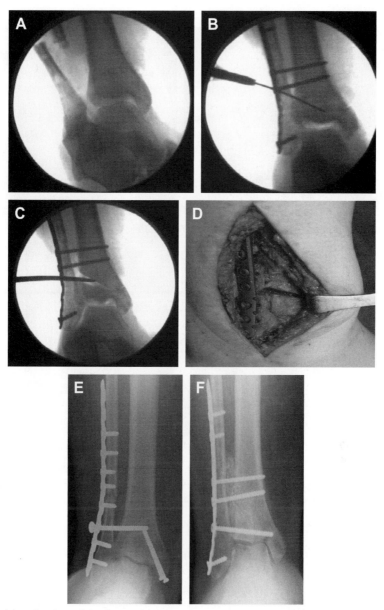

Fig. 8. (*A*) Reflection of the fibula. (*B*) Guide wire insertion for osteotomy planning (in this case the fibula was fixed out to length first). (*C*) Gentle step-wise opening of the osteotomy. (*D*) Insertion of bone graft wedge. (*E, F*) Preoperative malunion.

osteotomy (see earlier in this article). This is planned fluoroscopically using a K-wire inserted under vision. The first three fourths of the osteotomy is made with a saw along the plane of the guide pin, and the tibialis posterior tendon must be retracted, which is at risk throughout the osteotomy. The osteotomy is completed using an osteotome, which can be used to lever the site open the required amount. We no longer pre-drill

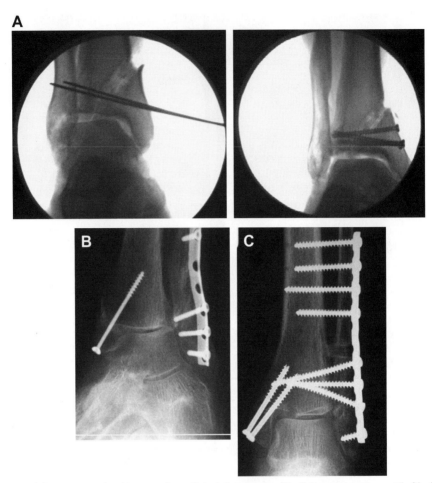

Fig. 9. (*A*) Intraoperative images of medial plafondplasty. (*B, C*) Reconstruction with fibula lengthening and de-rotation, syndesmosis stabilization, and medial malleolar corrective osteotomy.

the medial malleolus and use transverse screws or a plate to reduce the risk of a proximal shear (**Fig. 9**B,C).

Posterior Malleolar Malunion

Posterior malleolar malunion is an uncommon problem, and is often associated with a posterolateral subluxation of the talus in a complex trimalleolar fracture. The largest series in the recent literature by Weber and Ganz[12] describes four cases of malunion in just this scenario: the posterior fragments involved 27% to 40% of the articular surfaces, which were treated with osteotomy at up to 12 months post-injury. The approach used was a posterolateral one that was developed between the flexor hallucis longus and the peroneal tendons. On occasion a posteromedial approach was also required to mobilize the fragment after the periosteum was extensively released and it was still not free to swing on the attached posterior tibiofibular ligament and capsule.

A variety of fixation techniques were used including two anteroposterior screws and also a posterior antiglide plate. Weber and Ganz[12] recommended that when posterolateral instability of the talus occurred in the presence of a posterior malleolar malunion then this needed to be addressed, as lateral malleolar correction on its own would be insufficient. They noted that lateral joint space narrowing was not necessarily a result of cartilage loss and that posterolateral instability should be considered (**Fig. 10**).

Extra-Articular Deformity

Supramalleolar osteotomy is a useful procedure in the management of patients with extra-articular deformity regardless of the presence of marked degeneration. Even if the resolution of symptoms is short-lived or incomplete, the ankle is aligned well enough for ankle arthroplasty or arthrodesis. Excellent clinical results have been shown with both closing wedge (**Fig. 11A**) and opening wedge osteotomies.[13,14] Patients obtained significant pain relief and over short- to mid-term follow-up few showed radiographic evidence of progression of degeneration. Medial opening-wedge osteotomies have the advantage of being easier to perform and avoid shortening of the limb, but they take slightly longer to heal so the fixation and rehabilitation programs need to take this into account. Lateral closing-wedge osteotomies on the other hand are much more stable and so are easy to fix, do not need grafting, and eal reliably and rapidly. However, they necessitate a fibular osteotomy as well and result in some shortening of the limb (which will be 2 cm shorter than for an opening wedge osteotomy) and it weakens the peroneal muscles. Both procedures reliably correct the malalignment. In both techniques it is ideal to perform the osteotomy through the center of rotation and angulation (CORA). Correction at this point will produce anatomic realignment of the foot and ankle; however, this is not always feasible especially if it is too low. Correction elsewhere will translate the center of the ankle away from the mechanical axis and produce a zig-zag deformity. To prevent this, the distal tibia needs to be translated as well as angulated. The amount of correction clearly depends on the degree of deformity although some authors have advocated an

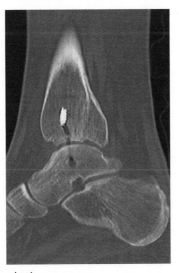

Fig. 10. Posterior malleolar malunion.

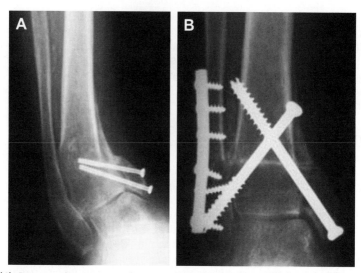

Fig. 11. (*A*) Preoperative varus malunion. Note the vessel calcification that necessitated closing wedge osteotomy instead of an opening wedge. (*B*) Postoperative closing wedge osteotomy.

overcorrection. The subtalar joint provides an important compensation for coronal plane stiffness at the ankle and therefore if this is stiff or angled itself then a biplanar calcaneal osteotomy may be required.

Stamatis and colleagues[15] described a technique for medial opening wedge osteotomy using a double approach. They advocated performing the medial osteotomy first, as the intact fibula provides useful stability and counterpressure when the tibial osteotomy is being opened with the laminar spreader. The tibia is exposed with an anteromedial incision, the saw cut can be planned using a guide wire as described earlier, and biplanar correction can be achieved by altering the angle of the saw blade in the sagittal plane. Ideally this should start at the CORA, if this is not possible then it should be through metaphyseal bone 4 to 5 cm proximal to the medial malleolus. A peri-articular locking plate is placed onto the bone to ensure that it permits adequate distal fixation of at least three screws. The osteotomy is then performed and opened using an osteotome and blunt laminar spreader. If translation is also required then the osteotomy is made through both cortices. The fibula osteotomy is made from the lateral side at the same level; this does not required fixation. Structural allograft is used to support the medial side.

The closing wedge osteotomy technique of Harstall and colleagues[13] is performed through a lateral approach to the fibula. The anterior soft tissues are elevated from the fibula and the tibia, preserving the periosteum. The posterior dissection requires incision of the peroneal fascia along the posterior border of the fibula. The peroneals are retracted exposing the fascia overlying the flexor hallucis longus. The posterior compartment is entered by elevating the fascia and the muscle fibers of the flexor hallucis longus off the fibula. The muscle attachments to the interosseous membrane and posterior tibia are bluntly elevated to give 2-cm access to the posteromedial cortex of the tibia. The peroneal vessels are at risk and need to be protected. The soft tissues are retracted anteriorly and posteriorly using Hohmann retractors and a guide wire is passed into the tibia in front of the fibula under fluoroscopic control to mark the osteotomy. This should be parallel to the

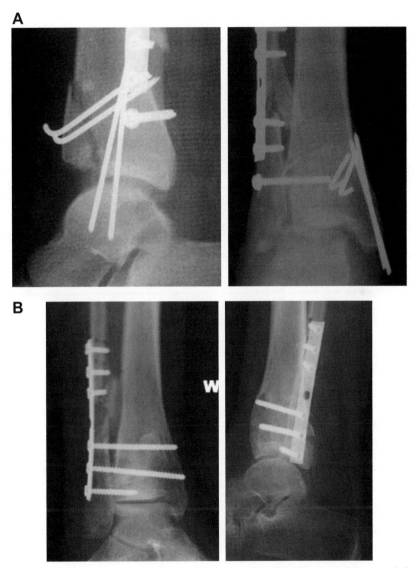

Fig. 12. (*A*) Complex malunion—deformity of the anterior tibia, fibula, and lateral plafond. (*B*) Correction with fibula lengthening and rotation, lateral plafondplasty, anterior tibial fixation, and syndesmosis stabilization.

joint surface and 3 cm above it; when making the osteotomy it is important to ensure that it is parallel to the joint line on the lateral view. The osteotomy is made with a saw blade that stops just lateral to the medial cortex. A second osteotomy is made to remove a wedge of bone the base of which is determined preoperatively and is approximately 1 mm per 1 degree of correction, although this can be accurately determined using the tangent of the correction angle.[16] Again this should stop short of the medial cortex. The osteotomy can then be hinged closed and fixed as shown in **Fig. 11**B.

SUMMARY

The aim of reconstructive surgery for an ankle malunion is joint preservation. The functional demands of the patient and the nature of the malunion need to be considered, but even in the presence of marked degeneration the patient may benefit from reasonable pain relief. Furthermore, deformity correction may be necessary to enable successful salvage surgery whether that is ankle fusion or arthroplasty. CT scanning can be a useful adjunct to plain radiography in assessing syndesmosis reduction and fibula rotation and consideration should be given to evaluation of the joint surface, as an osteochondral injury or loose bodies may compromise the results of the best reconstructions.

The malunion must be carefully evaluated to determine the direction and magnitude of each deformity—more than one may be present and each will need to be corrected using the techniques discussed (**Fig. 12**A,B). Operative planning will be based on this, although it must also take into account the nature of the soft tissues, pathology elsewhere in the foot, previous surgery, and future management.

REFERENCES

1. Wailing AK, SR. Ankle fractures in surgery of the foot and ankle. In: MR, Coughlin M, Saltzman C, editors. Surgery of the foot and ankle. Philadelphia: Elsevier; 2007. p. 1973.
2. Tunturi T, Kemppainen K, Patiala H, et al. Importance of anatomical reduction for subjective recovery after ankle fracture. Acta Orthop Scand 1983;54(4):641–7.
3. Moody ML, KJ, Hettinger E, et al. The effects of fibula and talar displacement on joint contact areas about the ankle. Orthop Rev 1992;21(6):741–4.
4. Offierski CM, GJ, Hall JH, et al. Late revision of fibular malunion in ankle fractures. Clin Orthop Relat Res 1982;171:145–9.
5. Singh R, AA, Davies M. Results of early surgical intervention after suboptimal ankle fracture fixation. Injury 2006;37(9):899–904.
6. Kelikian AS, KH. Aspects of tibial malleolar fractures. In: K, AS, editors. Disorders of the ankle. Philadelphia: WB Saunders; 1985.
7. Marti RK, RE, Nolte PA. Malunited ankle fractures. The late results of reconstruction. J Bone Joint Surg Br 1990;72(4):709–13.
8. Yablon IG, Leach RE. Reconstruction of malunited fractures of the lateral malleolus. J Bone Joint Surg Am 1989;71(4):521–7.
9. Panchbhavi VK, MM, Mason WT. Combination of hook plate and tibial pro-fibular screw fixation of osteoporotic fractures: a clinical evaluation of operative strategy. Foot Ankle Int 2005;26(7):510–5.
10. Ramsey PL, Hamilton W. Changes in tibiotalar area of contact caused by lateral talar shift. J Bone Joint Surg Am 1976;58:356–7.
11. Harper MC. Delayed reduction and stabilisation of the tibiofibular syndesmosis. Foot Ankle Int 2001;22(1):15–8.
12. Weber M, Ganz R. Malunion following trimalleolar fracture with posterolateral subluxation of the talus—reconstruction including the posterio malleolus. Foot Ankle Int 2003;24(4):338–44.
13. Harstall R, Lehmann O, Krause F, et al. Supramalleolar lateral closing wedge osteotomy for the treatment of varus ankle arthrosis. Foot Ankle Int 2007;28(5):542–8.
14. Stamatis ED, Cooper PS, Myerson MS. Supramalleolar osteotomy for the treatment of distal tibial angular deformities and arthritis of the ankle joint. Foot Ankle Int 2003;24:754–64.

15. Stamatis ED, Myerson MS. Supramalleolar osteotomy: indications and technique. Foot Ankle Clini N Am 2003;8(2):317–33.
16. Canale ST, Harper MC. Biotrigonometric analysis and practical applications of osteotomies of tibia in children. Instr Course Lect 1981;30:85–101.
17. McDaniel WJ, Wilson FC. Trimalleolar fractures of the ankle. An end result study. Clin Orthop 1977;122:37–45.
18. Mont MA, Sedlin ED, Weiner LS, et al. Postoperative radiographs as predictors of clinical outcome in unstable ankle fractures. J Orthop Trauma 1992;6(3):352–7.
19. Xenos JS, Hopkinson WJ, Mulligan ME, et al. The tibiofibular syndesmosis. Evaluation of the ligamentous structures, methods of fixation, and radiographic assessment. J Bone Joint Surg Am 1995;77(6):847–56.
20. Gardner MJ, Demtrakopoulos D, Briggs SM, et al. Malreduction of the tibiofibular syndesmosis in ankle fractures. Foot Ankle Int 2006;27(10):788–92.
21. Rolfe B, Nordt W, Sallis JG, et al. Assessing fibula length using bimalleolar angular measurements. Foot Ankle 1989;10(2):104–9.
22. Thordarsson DB, Motamed S, Hedman T, et al. The effect of fibular malreduction on contact pressures in an ankle fracture malunion model. J Bone Joint Surg Am 1997;79(12):1809–15.
23. Vasarhelyi A, Lubitz J, Gierer P, et al. Detection of fibular torsional deformities after surgery for ankle fractures with a novel CT method. Foot Ankle Int 2006; 27(12):1115–21.

Posttraumatic Avascular Necrosis of the Talus

Stephane Léduc, MD[a],*, Michael P. Clare, MD[b],
G. Yves Laflamme, MD[a], Arthur K. Walling, MD[b]

KEYWORDS

- Osteonecrosis • Avascular necrosis • Talus • Posttraumatic
- Traumatic • Joint-sparing • Joint-sacrificing

Avascular necrosis (AVN) of the talus is one the most challenging problems encountered in posttraumatic reconstruction of the hindfoot. Since the first description of the talus injury in 1608 by Fabricius of Hilden,[1] our knowledge of the talar anatomy, injuries, sequelae, and management has increased significantly. Adequate knowledge of the etiology, the extent of the disease, and the degree of patient symptoms are required to determine optimal treatment.

Talar osteonecrosis occurs when the vascular supply to the talus is interrupted and the bone is deprived of its oxygen source. Avascular necrosis of the talus can be isolated or associated with bone loss, collapse, sepsis, deformity, and severe arthritis of adjacent joints. Surgical alternatives include joint-sacrificing and joint-sparing procedures. Reconstructive procedures include isolated or extended fusions, osteotomies, bone grafting, soft tissues release, and joint replacement, alone or in combination; amputation remains a salvage option as well.

ANATOMY OF THE TALUS

The talus is the second largest tarsal bone and has a unique anatomy. Sixty percent of its surface is covered by articular cartilage and there are no muscular or tendinous attachments to the bone.[2,3] The inherent vascular supply of the talus is tenuous and, thus, predisposes it to avascular necrosis. The talus is characterized by extra-osseous arterial sources and variable intra-osseous blood supply. The extra-osseous vascularity is through the branches of the posterior tibial artery, the dorsalis pedis artery, and the perforating peroneal artery, which enter through nonarticulating surfaces of the bone.

---

[a] Department of Orthopaedic Surgery, Université de Montréal, Hôpital Sacré-Cœur de Montréal, 5400, boul. Gouin Ouest, Québec, Montréal, Canada, H4J 1C5
[b] Florida Orthopaedic Institute, 13020 Telecom Parkway N., Tampa, FL 33637, USA
* Corresponding author.
E-mail address: stephaneleduc@hotmail.com (S. Léduc).

Foot Ankle Clin N Am 13 (2008) 753–765
doi:10.1016/j.fcl.2008.09.004
1083-7515/08/$ – see front matter © 2008 Elsevier Inc. All rights reserved.

foot.theclinics.com

The major blood supply to the talar body is provided by the artery of the tarsal canal. The tarsal canal artery supplies the central and lateral two-thirds of the talar body. Deltoid branches arising from this artery supply the remaining medial third of the talar body.[4] Branches of the anterior tibial artery supply the superomedial half of the talar head and neck. The inferolateral half of the talar head and neck are supplied by the tarsal sinus artery and or the lateral tarsal artery. The intra-osseous anastomoses are variable among individuals and may explain why some patients develop AVN and while others do not.

CLASSIFICATION, ETIOLOGY, AND EPIDEMIOLOGY OF TALAR INJURY

In 1919, Anderson reported 18 cases of talus fracture in aviators.[5] Anderson identified the mechanism of injury as a hyperdorsiflexion force exerted on the sole of the foot by the rudder bar of the aircraft on impact, and coined the term "aviator's astragalus" for this injury because of its occurrence in belly landings of small aircraft. More recent reports[6–8] have described direct impact—a combination of axial and dorsiflexion energy—with the foot in inversion or eversion to explain the injury.

The risk of AVN of the talus is related to the degree of displacement of the injury and the resultant damage to the vascular component supplying the talus.[9,10] Hawkins[9] developed a classification in 1970 for vertical fractures of the talar neck, which was later modified by Canale and Kelly:[11] a Hawkins type 1 is a nondisplaced talar neck fracture and has 0% to 15% AVN risk; a Hawkins type 2 is a talar neck fracture associated with a subluxation or a dislocation of the subtalar joint and has a 20% to 50% AVN risk; a Hawkins type 3 is a talar neck fracture associated with subluxation or dislocation of the subtalar and ankle joint and has a 90% AVN risk; a Hawkins type 4 is a talar neck fracture associated with subluxation or dislocation of the subtalar, ankle, and talonavicular joints and has a 100% AVN risk. Patients in these series were treated with closed reduction and casting or primitive internal fixation techniques, which may have contributed to AVN rates. AVN rates from more recent series using modern internal fixation techniques have been substantially lower.[12,13]

The Marti-Weber classification has gained popularity for its inclusion of all talus injuries and its prognostic value with regard to AVN.[14] Type I injuries include lateral process fractures, posterior process fractures, osteochondral flake fractures, and talus head with very distal neck fractures, none of which are associated with the development of AVN. Type II injuries include vertical fractures of the proximal neck or talar body without displacement, in which AVN is rarely seen. Type III injuries are type II injuries with displacement plus dislocation or subluxation of the subtalar or ankle joint, which are typically associated with AVN. Type IV injuries include a neck or body fracture with complete talar body dislocation from both the subtalar and the ankle joints, which are almost always associated with AVN.

Inokuchi and colleagues[15] found that the vertical fracture of the talus that extends inferiorly in the posterior facet of the talus is a talar body fracture with a higher prevalence of AVN, and a worse prognosis than a vertical talar body fracture not involving the posterior facet. Recent studies[12,13] have shown that a delay in surgical fixation does not appear to affect the outcome, union, or prevalence of osteonecrosis.

CLINICAL INVESTIGATION

Posttraumatic sequelae of talus injury are common and include chronic pain, stiffness, or loss of function. Adequate evaluation as to the personality of the disease is needed. A thorough clinical and physical evaluation is crucial. Clinical and physical assessment includes type of pain, local or systemic signs of infection, and assessment of deformity, motion, soft-tissue quality, and neurovascular examination. If infection is suspected, C-reactive protein, sedimentation rate, and nuclear medicine should be obtained.

RADIOLOGIC ASSESSMENT OF TALUS AVN

Plain radiography remains the primary diagnostic tool for AVN of the talus; however, CT scanning and MRI provide additional insight in delineating subtle disease and to more thoroughly evaluate deformity and adjacent sequela.[16] Plain radiographs and CT scans can help identify the presence of arthritic changes, bone loss, bone quality, and deformity. Selective injections can assist in distinguishing pain sources in the ankle joint, subtalar joint, talonavicular joint, or combinations thereof.

Plain Radiology

Initially, the necrotic bone and surrounding viable bone are equal in opacity. Over time, local hyperemia promotes the resorption of healthy bone, making the viable bone appear osteopenic. Conversely, the lack of blood supply in necrotic bone prevents its resorption, making necrotic bone appear more radiopaque than the surrounding osteopenic bone. At this point, radiographic evidence of talar AVN becomes obvious. With time, reossification of the necrotic bone occurs and increases its sclerotic appearance.[17]

AVN is diagnosed on plain radiography by the absence of the Hawkins sign.[9] The Hawkins sign is a radiolucent band in the talar dome that is indicative of viability and typically appears at 6 to 8 weeks following a talus fracture (**Fig. 1**). Tezval and colleagues[18] found that the presence of the Hawkins sign is an excellent predictor of vascularity of the talus after a talus fracture. If a full or partial Hawkins sign is detected, it is unlikely that AVN will occur. However, the absence of the Hawkins sign does not reliably correlate with AVN of the talus; in their series, the presence of a Hawkins sign had a sensitivity of 100% and specificity of 57.7%.

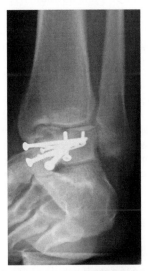

Fig. 1. Hawkins sign in a 20-year-old female who had undergone open reduction internal fixation for injuries sustained in a car accident. Radiograph (mortice view) shows a thin subchondral area of radiolucency involving the entire talar dome (positive Hawkins sign), a finding that signifies talar viability and excludes future development of AVN.

CT Scan and MRI

CT Scan also reveals characteristic talar AVN patterns and can be used to confirm radiographic findings. It helps to assess subtle depression, collapse, fragmentation, and arthritic changes. MRI is the most sensitive technique for detecting osteonecrosis of the talus, especially in the early stages.[19]

CONSERVATIVE TREATMENT

The presence of AVN of the talus before collapse is initially managed nonoperatively. Creeping substitution of the talus body can require 36 months to occur. Some investigators, including Hawkins, advocated extended nonweight-bearing;[20–22] Canale recommended nonweight-bearing until revascularization is obtained.[21] Other investigators have recommended a patellar tendon-bearing brace until reconstitution of the talar body is complete.[23–25] However, patient compliance is rarely possible for 36 months.[26] Penny and colleagues[27] showed that weight-bearing on a sclerotic and avascular talus poses no real danger for dome collapse, and found no correlation between poor results with AVN of the talus and time of nonweight-bearing.[27] The current trend is to permit weight-bearing as tolerated.

CORE DECOMPRESSION

Core decompression has been suggested as an alternative for treatment of nontraumatic AVN of the talus without collapse by decreasing intra-osseous pressure and enhancing revascularization. Mont and colleagues[28] concluded that core decompression is a viable method of treatment for symptomatic avascular necrosis of the talus before collapse. At 7 years, 82% of the 17 ankles treated by core decompression had excellent or good result. Delanois and colleagues[29] also supported core decompression in symptomatic atraumatic AVN of the talus before collapse. They reported fair-to-excellent results in 29 of 32 patients with AVN of the talus without collapse treated with core decompression.

SURGICAL RECONSTRUCTION OF A NONINFECTED TALUS AVN WITH COLLAPSE

Several treatment options are available for a patient who has pain and disability associated with isolated or combined arthrosis of the ankle, subtalar, talonavicular joint, and osteonecrosis of the body of the talus. These options include joint-sacrificing and joint-sparing procedures. Joint-sacrificing options include resection of the talar body with or without tibiocalcaneal arthrodesis, conventional resection of the joint and arthrodesis, arthrodesis with use of an anterior-sliding tibial bone graft, and posterior tibiotalocalcaneal arthrodesis. Joint-sparing procedures include standard or custom-made total ankle replacement, nonvascularized allograft, and vascularized autograft.

JOINT-SACRIFICING PROCEDURES
Total Talectomy

Simple subtotal or total talectomy without fusion has historically been met with poor results, as almost all patients have a residually painful foot.[9,30–33] More recently, Marsh and colleagues[34] presented two patients with three talectomies performed at 4 and 10 months after injury for infection. Favorable results were reported at follow-up of 21 and 14 years, respectively.

Arthrodesis

Principles of arthrodesis

Successful arthrodesis will improve the patient function but will still be disabling. Preparation of the fusion site requires removal of cartilage and necrotic bone to provide a viable bleeding bone surface for fusion. The fusion site may need bone grafting to fill smaller defects; structural grafting may be necessary for larger defects. Successful fusion depends on stable, rigid fixation achieved by screws, or plate and screws; alternatively, fixation may be obtained with a nail or external fixation. Absence of sufficient bone may preclude an isolated arthrodesis and may thus require extending the fusion to multiple joints. The primary goal is to recreate a plantigrade foot.

Ankle arthrodesis

Ankle arthrodesis is a reliable alternative for AVN of the talus with collapse in cases where symptoms are isolated to the ankle joint. Sufficient talus bone stock following debridement of the AVN is required for adequate fixation of the ankle joint. Structural defects of the talus are filled with a structural autograft or allograft. Kitaoka and Patzer[35] reported reliable results after arthrodesis for talar AVN in 19 patients; 3 had an isolated ankle fusion and 16 had a combined ankle and subtalar fusion.

Standard fixation for ankle arthrodesis includes multiplanar screws or plate fixation. Tarkin and colleagues showed that compared with screws alone, anterior plate supplementation increases construct rigidity and decreases micromotion at the ankle-fusion interface.[36] A preliminary clinical study reported a union rate of 96% with anterior plate supplementation.[37] External fixation has also been used to achieve an ankle fusion.[38] Antegrade nailing of the ankle joint has been described, but with suboptimal results because of bad fixation in the talus. Retrograde nailing is not recommanded because it violates the subtalar joint. Because the success of ankle arthrodesis depends on achieving and maintaining rigid fixation of the prepared tibiotalar interface, the authors recommend fixation with screws and anterior plate supplementation (**Fig. 2**).

Subtalar fusion

Subtalar arthrodesis is a reliable alternative for AVN of the talus with an intact talar dome where symptoms are isolated to the subtalar joint, which is uncommon. After adequate debridement, restoration of the anatomy of the hindfoot may require

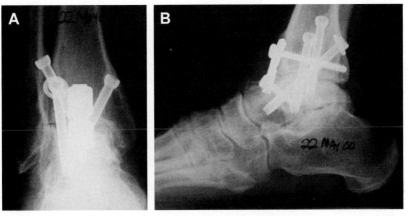

Fig. 2. Postoperative AP (*A*) and lateral (*B*) radiographs of an ankle arthrodesis performed with a combination of screws supplemented with an anterior plate.

a structural bone graft. Rigid fixation of the subtalar joint is achieved by standard (large fragment) cancellous screws or cannulated screws. Sufficient talus bone after debridement of the AVN is similarly required for adequate fixation of the subtalar joint.

Talonavicular fusion

Isolated talonavicular joint symptoms are still preferably treated by talonavicular fusion than by a triple arthrodesis. After adequate debridement, restoration of the anatomy of the medial column may require a structural bone graft. Standard fixation of the talonavicular joint requires screws (small fragment 3.5-mm or 4.0-mm cancellous). A small or minifragment plate or staples can be used to supplement the fixation construct where necessary.

Blair tibiotalar fusion

Blair fusion involves removal of the talar body with maintenance of the talar neck and head. The distal anterior tibia is then fused with the remaining talus. Some have modified the initial technique by adding a structural graft anteriorly or by adding fixation devices. The advantages of the Blair fusion compared with a tibiocalcaneal arthrodesis include the preservation of some hindfoot motion, less limb shortening, and a relatively normal looking foot. However, unfavorable results have been reported by Morris and colleagues,[39] Canale and Kelly,[11] and Dennis and Tullos.[40] Most recently, Marsh and colleagues[34] presented one case of Blair fusion for osteomyelitis 9 months after injury, with an excellent result.

Tibiocalcaneal fusion and tibiotalocalcaneal fusion

Removal of the entire talar body will necessitate a double-hindfoot fusion. Maintenance of limb length and foot shape aid in fitting shoe wear. Double fusion without structural grafting has fallen out of favor because it shortens the leg.[41,42] Reckling[42] described a technique whereby a subtotal or total talectomy with resection of both malleoli was performed to allow the cut surfaces of the distal tibia and the calcaneus to fuse.

Tibiotalocalcaneal (TTC) fusions can be accomplished using cancellous screws, cannulated screws (**Fig. 3**),[41,43] plates and screws, intramedullary nails (**Fig. 4**),[44] external fixation,[45,46] and free vascularized fibula grafts. Kile and colleagues[44] reported on the use of a retrograde femoral supracondylar nail to stabilize an extra-articular construct in 30 consecutive patients, including 3 patients with AVN of the talus. Using

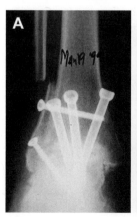
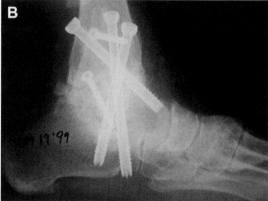

Fig. 3. Postoperative AP (*A*) and lateral (*B*) radiographs of a successful double hindfoot fusion with cannulated screws.

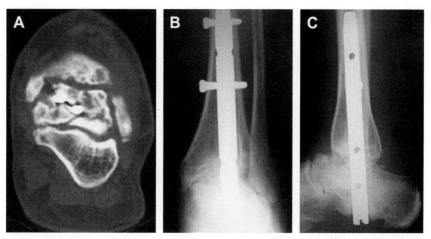

Fig. 4. Preoperative coronal CT scan (*A*) of a posttraumatic AVN of the talus involving the ankle and subtalar joint. Postoperative AP (*B*) and lateral (*C*) of a successful double hindfoot fusion with hindfoot nail.

anterior plate techniques, Sanders and colleagues[47] were able to obtain a 100% fusion rate in a series of 11 patients who required TTC or pantalar fusion for severe grade IIIB open-tibial pilon and talus fractures. Options to fill the defect include tricortical iliac crest autograft, structural allograft, or femoral head allograft.[48]

Triple and pantalar arthrodesis
When the subtalar and talonavicular joints are involved, triple arthrodesis is required. Involvement of the ankle, subtalar and talonavicular joints necessitates a pantalar fusion.

JOINT-SPARING PROCEDURE

Impaired residual function and the development of adjacent joint arthritis following fusion have prompted surgeons to look for joint-sparing alternatives. Bone substitutes or joint replacement for AVN of the talus are promising new techniques.

Allograft Reconstruction
AVN of the talus involving only the talar dome with ankle arthritis can be addressed with fresh osteochondral total ankle allograft transplantation. Gross and colleagues[49] reported nine cases of osteochondral defects of the talus treated with fresh osteochondral allograft transplantation. Eight patients had osteochondritis dissecans and one had an open talus fracture. All underwent partial talar allograft transplantation and the survival rate at 11 years was six out of nine patients. When the talar AVN is associated with collapse and ankle arthritis, allograft total ankle replacement is an alternative. Jeng and Myerson[50] described 29 patients that underwent bipolar osteochondral allograft of the ankle joint, including 2 patients with talar AVN treated, and had a 50% success rate (**Fig. 5**). There are no long-term results for talar allograft survival rates in larger cohorts or studies; there are currently no data on revascularization, which is considered to be the most important factor for remodeling of the talus.

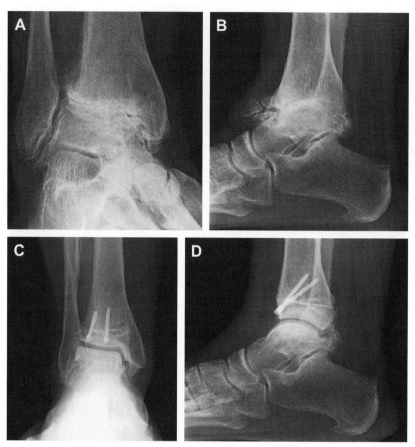

Fig. 5. Preoperative AP (*A*) and lateral (*B*) radiographs of a patient with ankle arthritis secondary to a talar AVN. Postoperative AP (*C*) and lateral (*D*) radiographs of the same patient following a successful fresh osteochondral total ankle allograft transplantation. (*Courtesy of* Mark Myerson, MD, Baltimore, Maryland.)

Vascularized Autograft Reconstruction

Successful treatment of AVN of the femoral head with a fibula vascularized graft has encouraged some surgeons to apply the same concepts to the talus. In 1989, Hussl and colleagues[51] reported use of a vascularized bone graft from the iliac crest for revascularization of the talus in posttraumatic AVN in a 16-year-old patient. In 2001, Gilbert and colleagues[52] studied 14 fresh-frozen cadaver lower extremities and were able to identify a consistent blood supply to the distal fibula, cuboid, and cuneiform I and III with reliable nutrient arteries. Zhang and colleagues[53] reported on the curative effect of vascularized bone graft in the treatment of 24 AVNs of the talus, with a success rate of 83.3% at 3 to 5 years follow-up. Horst and colleagues[54] have reported the use of this technique as well but without results yet.

Joint Replacement

Joint replacement is an alternative to fusion but currently without knowledge of long-term outcome (**Fig. 6**). Joint replacement requires a stable and solid bony surface to support the implant over time. Complete debridement of the AVN will often prevent

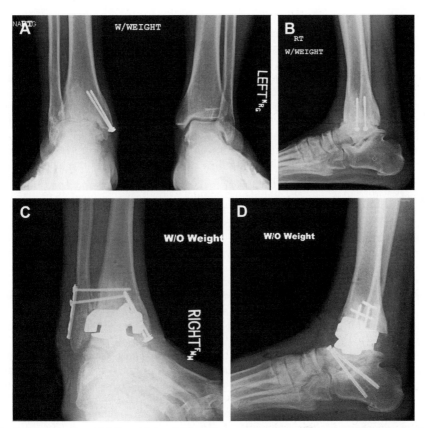

Fig. 6. Preoperative AP (*A*) and lateral (*B*) radiographs of a patient with ankle and subtalar arthritis secondary to a talar AVN. Postoperative AP (*C*) and lateral (*D*) radiographs of the same patient following a successful total ankle replacement combined with a subtalar fusion. (*Courtesy of* Mark Myerson, MD, Baltimore, Maryland.)

a standard tibiotalar replacement. A customized talar component can be ordered to address the defect and even replace the talar body completely. Harnroongroj and colleagues[55] published satisfactory results of talar body prosthetic replacement in 14 of 16 patients in Thailand, with average follow-up of 9.5 years. Currently, however, there are no other long-term results available for ankle arthroplasty in these, often, young patients.

SURGICAL RECONSTRUCTION OF AN INFECTED AVN OF THE TALUS

Salvage of an infected AVN of the talus has to be addressed similar to an unstable infected nonunion in that it presents two difficult problems: osteomyelitis and nonunion. Simultaneous treatment of each can be difficult or impossible because the treatment of one can negatively influence the treatment of the other. In general, a fusion requires stability to promote union of the bone interfaces, typically provided in the form of metal implants. Metal implants, however, promote both adherence of microbes and biofilm formation, and adversely affects phagocytosis, thereby making eradication of infection more difficult.[56,57]

The successful treatment of infected talar AVN should include a multidisciplinary approach designed to treat each component of the problem while taking into consideration confounding patient factors. Therefore, the authors favor a two-stage protocol, with the initial stage consisting of removal of all implants, aggressive debridement and irrigation, temporary stabilization of the defect, prevention of dead-space formation, and bacterial-specific antibiotic treatment. To prevent any resultant dead space being filled by unwanted tissue or fluid collection, and to help local administration of antibiotic, an antibiotic-impregnated cement block can be placed within the defect. The antibiotic-impregnated polymethyl methacrylate (PMMA) delivers high local concentrations of antibiotics and maintains space for later bone grafting. A PMMA block can reduce soft tissue in-growth, augment the local stability, and maintain length and space for the later reconstruction stage of the treatment (**Fig. 7**).

To provide a mechanically stable environment without internal implants requires either the use of an external fixator or a cast. Medical management of the infection includes administration of local and systemic antibiotics. In collaboration with an infectious disease specialist, appropriate selection and duration of intravenous antibiotic administration is based upon the type of bacteria found at the infection site and the quality of the host.[58] After 6 weeks of antibiotic treatment, confirmation that the infection has been eradicated can be made with some degree of certainty with physical examination, laboratory tests (erythrocyte sedimentation rate, C-reactive protein), and a biopsy of the area. A culture-negative biopsy taken after antibiotics have been discontinued for at least 5 to 7 days will also support that the infection has been eradicated.

At that time, definitive reconstruction of the talus can safely be performed. Optimizing the treatment of infection also includes optimal control of the immunologic and healing process, which includes careful control of blood glucose levels and patient nutrition. The second stage is initiated once the infection has been eradicated and includes fusion, as described above. Joint-sparing procedures are not recommended in a previously infected environment.

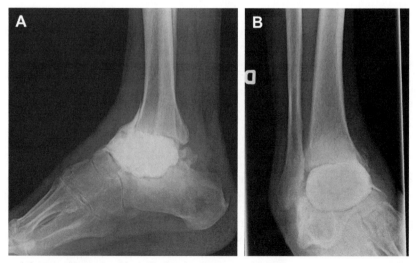

Fig. 7. (*A*) AP and lateral ankle radiodraphs showing a (*B*) PMMA cement block used during stage 1 of a salvage of an infected posttraumatic AVN of the talus.

AMPUTATION

Salvage of a nonfunctional limb is not reasonable. Sanders and colleagues[47] raised the question of salvage versus amputation for complex and open hindfoot injuries. Amputation may be the better solution in certain situations.

SUMMARY

Avascular necrosis of the talus is one the most challenging problems encountered in posttraumatic reconstruction of the hindfoot. Adequate knowledge of the etiology, the extent of the disease, and the degree of patient symptoms are required to optimally treat this condition. If the patient has failed nonoperative treatment, then reconstruction or salvage is considered. These options include joint-sacrificing and joint-sparing procedures. Although there are many published treatments for posttraumatic AVN of the talus, critical outcome studies are still lacking.

REFERENCES

1. Bonnin JG. Dislocations and fracture dislocations of the talus. Br J Surg 1940;28: 88–100.
2. Kelly PJ, Sullivan CR. Blood supply of the talus. Clin Orthop 1963;30:37–44.
3. Berlet GC, Lee TH, Massa EG. Talar neck fractures. Orthop Clin North Am 2001; 32:53–64.
4. Gelberman RH, Mortensen WW. The arterial anatomy of the talus. Foot Ankle 1983;4:64–72.
5. Anderson HG. The medical and surgical aspects of aviation. London: Oxford University Press; 1919.
6. Sanders DW. Fractures of the talus; fractures in adults. In: Bucholz RW, Heckman JD, Court-Brown CM, editors. vol. 6. Philadelphia: Lippincott Williams and Wilkins; 2006. p. 2249–92.
7. Peterson L, Romanus B, Dahlberg E. Fracture of the collum talidan experimental study. J Biomech 1976;9(4):277–9.
8. Daniels TR, Smith JW. Foot fellow's review. Foot Ankle Int 1993;14:225–34.
9. Hawkins LG. Fractures of the neck of the talus. J Bone Joint Surg Am 1970;52(5): 991–1002.
10. Metzger MJ, Levin JS, Clancy JT. Talar neck fractures and rates of avascular necrosis. J Foot Ankle Surg 1999;38(2):154–62.
11. Canale ST, Kelly FB Jr. Fractures of the neck of the talus. J Bone Joint Surg Am 1978;60:143–56.
12. Lindvall E, Haidukewych G, Dispasquale T, et al. Open reduction and stable fixation of isolated, displaced talar neck and body fractures. J Bone Joint Surg Am 2004;86:2229–34.
13. Vallier HA, Nork SE, Benirschke SK, et al. Surgical treatment of talar body fractures. J Bone Joint Surg Am 2003;85:1716–24.
14. Marti R. Talus und Calcaneusfrakturen. In: Weber BG, Brunner C, Freuler F, editors. Die Frakturenbehandlung bei Kindern und Jugendlichen. Berlin: Springer-Verlag; 1978. p. 373–84 [In German].
15. Inokuchi S, Ogawa K, Usami N. Classification of fractures of the talus: clear differentiation between neck and body fractures. Foot Ankle Int 1996;17:748–50.
16. Pearce DH, Mongiardi CN, Fornasier VL, et al. Necrosis of the talus: a pictorial essay. Radiographics 2005;25:399–410.

17. Christman RA, Cohen R. Osteonecrosis and osteochondrosis. In: Foot and ankle radiology. St Louis (MO): Churchill Livingstone; 2003. p. 452–81.

18. Tezval M, Dumont C, Sturmer KM. Prognostic reliability of the Hawkins sign in fractures of the talus. J Orthop Trauma 2007;21(8):538–43.

19. Thordarson DB, Triffon MJ, Terk MR. Magnetic resonance imaging to detect avascular necrosis after open reduction and internal fixation of talar neck fractures. Foot Ankle Int 1996;17:742–7.

20. Adelaar RS. The treatment of complex fractures of the talus. Orthop Clin North Am 1989;20:691–707.

21. Canale ST. Fractures of the neck of the talus. Orthopedics 1990;10:1105–15.

22. Kenwright J, Taylor RG. Major injuries of the talus. J Bone Joint Surg Br 1970;52: 36–48.

23. Comfort TH, Behrens F, Gaither DW, et al. Long-term results of displaced talar neck fractures. Clin Orthop 1985;199:81–7.

24. Grob D, Simpson LA, Weber BG, et al. Operative treatment of displaced talus fractures. Clin Orthop 1985;199:88–96.

25. Szyszkowitz R, Reschauer R, Seggl W. Eighty-five talus fractures treated by ORIF with five to eight years of follow-up study of 69 patients. Clin Orthop 1985;199: 97–107.

26. Rammelt S, Zwipp H, Gavlik JM. Avascular necrosis after minimally displaced talus fracture in a child. Foot Ankle Int 2000;21:1030–6.

27. Penny JN, Davis LA. Fractures and fracture-dislocations of the neck of the talus. J Trauma 1980;20(12):1029–37.

28. Mont MA, Schon LC, Hungerford MW, et al. Avascular necrosis of the talus treated by core decompression. J Bone Joint Surg Am 1996;78:827–30.

29. Delanois RE, Mont MA, Yoon TR, et al. Atraumatic osteonecrosis of the talus. J Bone Joint Surg Am 1998;80:529–36.

30. Coltart WD. Aviator's astragalus. J Bone Joint Surg Br 1952;34:545–66.

31. McKeever FM. Treatment of complications of fractures and dislocations of the talus. Clin Orthop Relat Res 1963;30:45–52.

32. Dunn AR, Jacobs B, Campbell RD Jr. Fractures of the talus. J Trauma 1966;6(4): 443–68.

33. Pennal GF, Yadav MP. Operative treatment of comminuted fractures of the Os calcis. Orthop Clin North Am 1973;4(1):197–211.

34. Marsh JL, Saltzman CL, Iverson M, et al. Major open injuries of the talus. J Orthop Trauma 1995;9:371–6.

35. Kitaoka HB, Patzer GL. Arthrodesis for the treatment of arthrosis of the ankle and osteonecrosis of the talus. J Bone Joint Surg Am 1998;80(3):370–9.

36. Tarkin IS, Mormino MA, Clare MP, et al. Anterior plate supplementation increases ankle arthrodesis construct rigidity. Foot Ankle Int 2007;28(2): 219–23.

37. Steinlauf SD, Heir K, Walling A, et al. Anatomic compression arthrodesis technique (ACAT) for post traumatic arthrosis of the ankle. OTA Trans 2000. Available at: www.ota.org. Accessed October 20, 2008.

38. Johnson EE, Weltmer J, Lian GJ, et al. Ilizarov ankle arthrodesis. Clin Orthop Relat Res 1992;280:160–9.

39. Morris H, Hand W, Dunn W. The modified Blair fusion for fractures of the talus. J Bone Joint Surg Am 1971;53:1289–97.

40. Dennis MD, Tullos HS. Blair tibiotalar arthrodesis for injuries to the talus. J Bone Joint Surg Am 1980;62:103–7.

41. Mann RA, Chou LB. Tibiocalcaneal arthrodesis. Foot Ankle Int 1995;16:401–5.

42. Reckling FW. Early tibiocalcaneal fusion in the treatment of severe injuries of the talus. J Trauma 1972;12:390–6.

43. Papa JA, Myerson MS. Pantalar and tibiotalocalcaneal arthrodesis for posttraumatic osteoarthrosis of the ankle and hindfoot. J Bone Joint Surg Am 1992;74: 1042–9.

44. Kile TA, Donnelly RE, Gehrke JC, et al. Tibiotalocalcaneal arthrodesis with an intramedullary device. Foot Ankle Int 1994;15:669–73.

45. Johnson KA. Surgery of the foot and ankle. New York: Raven; 1989.

46. Russotti GM, Johnson KA, Cass JR. Tibiotalocalcaneal arthrodesis for arthritis and deformity of the hind part of the foot. J Bone Joint Surg Am 1988;70:1304–7.

47. Sanders R, Helfet DL, Pappas J, et al. The salvage of grade IIIB open ankle and talus fractures. J Orthop Trauma 1992;6:201–8.

48. Reed LR, Sanders RW. Use of bulk allografts in complex hindfoot reconstruction. La Jolla (CA): American Orthopaedic Foot and Ankle Society; 2006.

49. Gross AE, Agnidis Z, Hutchison CR. Osteochondral defects of the talus treated with fresh osteochondral allograft transplantation. Foot Ankle Int 2001;22:385–91.

50. Jeng CL, Kadakia A, White KL, et al. Fresh osteochondral total ankle allograft transplantation for the treatment of ankle arthritis. Foot Ankle Int 2008;29(6): 554–60.

51. Hussl H, Sailer R, Daniaux H, et al. Revascularization of a partially necrotic talus with a vascularized bone graft from the iliac crest. Arch Orthop Trauma Surg 1989;108:27–9.

52. Gilbert B, Horst F, Nunley J. Potential donor rotational bone grafts using vascular territories in the foot and ankle. J Bone Joint Surg Am 2004;86(9):1857–73.

53. Zhang Y, Liu Y, Jiang Y. Treatment of avascular necrosis of talus with vascularized bone graft. Zhongguo Xiu Fu Chong Jian Wai Ke Za Zhi 1998;12(5):285–7.

54. Horst F, Gilbert BJ, Nunley JA. Avascular necrosis of the talus: current treatment options. Foot Ankle Clin N Am 2004;9:757–73.

55. Harnroongroj T, Vanadurongwan V. The talar body prosthesis. J Bone Joint Surg Am 1997;79(9):1313–22.

56. Gristina AG. Biomaterial-centered infection: microbial adhesion versus tissue integration. Science 1987;237:1588–95.

57. Gristina AG, Naylor PT, Myrvik QN. Mechanisms of musculoskeletal sepsis. Orthop Clin North Am 1991;22:363–71.

58. Cierny G III, Mader JT, Penninck JJ. A clinical staging system for adult osteomyelitis. Clin Orthop 2003;414:7–24.

Salvage of Compartment Syndrome of the Leg and Foot

Jennifer M.B. Brey, MD[a], Michael D. Castro, DO[b],*

KEYWORDS

- Treatment • Late effects • Compartment syndrome
- Volkmann's contracture

Compartment syndrome occurs when the pressure within a contained area of tissue increases to a level high enough to cause damage to the structures within that space. While most often associated with fractures, compartment syndrome may be seen resulting from soft-tissue trauma, burns, and blood dyscrasias.

The diagnosis of compartment syndrome is most often made on a clinical basis. Pain with passive stretch of the muscles within the compartment is generally accepted as the most sensitive diagnostic indicator for compartment syndrome of the leg or foot. Symptoms associated with compartment syndrome of the foot may be masked by the pain due to the causative injury. Pain, parasthesias, changes in temperature and color, paralysis, and occasionally pulselessness are considered the hallmark findings of the disorder. For patients with low Glascow Coma Scores and decreased mentation, or for those in whom the symptoms are vague, the diagnosis may need to be made by direct measurement of compartment pressures. Unless there are complicating factors, compartment syndrome should be treated immediately to avoid irreversible damage to the contents of the affected limb.

In some cases, the diagnosis and treatment of compartment syndrome cannot be made in a rapid manner. Patients may be "found down" after several hours or days on an extremity resulting in vascular compromise and ischemia. Other patients who may not be able to communicate the above-mentioned symptoms may have a delay in care. Still others may be dismissed as problem patients seeking pain medication. Delay in treatment may be devastating to the patient, resulting in muscle necrosis, nerve damage, and risk of rhabdomyolysis. Late sequelae include ischemic

[a] Drexel College of Medicine, Department of Orthopaedic Surgery, 245 North 15th Street, MS 420,Philadelphia, PA 19102, USA
[b] The Center for Orthopaedic Research and Education, 3811 E Bell Road, Suite 302, Phoenix, AZ 85032, USA
* Corresponding author.
E-mail address: michael.castro@mac.com (M.D. Castro).

Foot Ankle Clin N Am 13 (2008) 767–772
doi:10.1016/j.fcl.2008.08.003
1083-7515/08/$ – see front matter © 2008 Elsevier Inc. All rights reserved.

foot.theclinics.com

contractures, chronic pain, and psychosocial and economic costs to the patient. The delay in diagnosis of compartment syndrome is noted to be a major source of litigation, with an average compensation of $426,000 per case in 2004.[1]

The sequelae of compartment syndrome are thought to be due to impairment of the microcirculation within the compartment. Bourne and Rorabeck studied the effects of magnitude and duration of pressure within the anterolateral compartment of the leg in a dog. They found that while blood flow to the injured extremity returns to normal within two hours of compartment release, the damage to other soft tissue structures was more permanent. The peroneal nerve, in particular, was especially more sensitive to prolonged pressure than the skeletal muscle. The slowing of the conduction velocity was dependent on both the magnitude and duration of increased pressure.[2] The degree of muscle damage due to compartment syndrome is dependent on both magnitude and duration as well. Damaged muscle may undergo necrosis for 6 to 12 months following ischemic injury. During this time, longitudinal and horizontal scar formation, and adhesion to surrounding tissues, cause muscle and tendon shortening and decreased tendon excursion. This may also lead to contracture and loss of motion of surrounding joints.[3]

The treatment of compartment syndrome of the leg is surgical decompression of all four compartments. This is usually done by a combined medial and lateral approach.[4] The medial incision is made just posterior to the tibia and will decompress the superficial and deep compartments of the leg. A lateral incision is made over the fibula and decompresses the anterior and lateral compartments, and may be used to release the superficial posterior compartment. The length of the incisions should be at least 16 cm to release pressure caused by the skin on compartment.[5] Damaged muscle is debrided as necessary, with a second debridement usually performed 36 to 72 hours after initial release.[6] The wounds are closed by gradual approximation or placement of skin grafts.

Compartment syndrome of the foot has also been described following crush injuries, forefoot and midfoot fractures, and calcaneal fractures.[7] Because of the communication between the deep posterior compartment of the leg and the calcaneal compartment of the foot, there is a theoretic risk of foot compartment syndrome after tibial fracture. Fakhouri and Manoli have reported on foot compartment syndrome following a tibial plateau fracture as well as leg compartment syndrome following multiple metatarsal fractures.[7] Bayer and colleagues[8] reported no chronic deformities of the foot following a series of 49 patients with tibial shaft fractures.

Manoli has identified nine compartments of the foot, with three running the entire length of the foot (medial, lateral, and superficial) as well as six localized compartments (four interossei compartments, the adductor, and the calcaneal).[9–11] The calcaneal compartment was found to contain the quadratus plantae muscle as well as the lateral plantar nerve. Andermahr and colleagues[12] have also found that in cases of sustentacular calcaneal fracture, bleeding into the calcaneal compartment may cause a severe increase in pressure that can lead to compression of the medial and lateral plantar arteries and nerves. However, they did find that the medial plantar structures are less prone to damage based on their location outside of the osteofibrous compartment.

Treatment of compartment syndrome of the foot, much like that of the leg, also consists of decompressive fasciotomy. A three incision technique is now accepted as the standard approach to the compartments of the foot. The hindfoot incision is made parallel to the heel pad of the foot a distance of approximately 6 cm on the medial surface. This approach will decompress the medial, superficial, calcaneal, and lateral compartments. Two dorsal incisions are made over the second and fourth metatarsal shafts that will decompress the four interosseus and adductor compartments.[9]

LATE EFFECTS

Deformities of the foot and ankle due to missed or undertreated compartment syndrome may be divided into extrinsic and intrinsic causes. Extrinsic deformities are due to injury mainly within the compartments of the leg. Conversely, intrinsic deformities are those due to injury of the soft tissue of the foot. The four compartments of the leg and nine compartments of the foot can each lead to their own specific deformities. The most common deformities include ankle equinus, equinovarus, foot cavus, and claw or hammertoes. Both neurologic injury and muscle contracture can contribute to the deformities.

Extrinsic deformities of the foot are most likely observed after fractures of the tibia. Deformities associated with leg compartment syndrome include clawtoes, hammertoes, equinus, equinovarus, cavus, pes planus, and abduction.[13] Cavus deformities of the foot result from damage to the muscles of the deep posterior compartment of the leg or tibial nerve injury. The contracture of the tibialis posterior muscle causes medial and dorsal subluxation of the talonavicular joint.[3] Equinus and equinovarus deformities of the foot may result from damage to structures within the superficial posterior compartment of the leg. Varus deformity may result from either contracture of the gastrocsoleus complex in the superficial compartment or overpull of the tibialis posterior muscle or extrinsic toe flexors in the deep compartment.[3,13] Toe deformities resulting from compartment syndrome of the leg may be due to contractures of the deep posterior and anterior compartments. This leads to clawing of the toes due to overpull of both flexors and extensors, with flexion of the DIP and PIP joints and extension of the MTP joints.

Karlström and colleagues[13] described 23 cases of foot and ankle deformity after tibial shaft fracture. Thirteen patients had clawing of the great toe, while 18 had hammertoe deformities. They also found a decreased distance from the lateral malleolus to the Achilles tendon, which they suggested was due to dorsiflexion of the talocrural joint.

Intrinsic deformities are due to soft tissue injuries within the compartments of the foot. The deformities most associated with contractures in this area are hammertoes and clawtoes. Clawtoe and hammertoe deformity can result from injury to the interosseous and lumbrical muscles of the forefoot. Contracture of the quadratus plantae muscle due to necrosis causes additional deformity due to its insertion on the extrinsic toe flexors.[13] Neurologic deficiency and chronic pain may be due to injury of the posterior tibial nerve as it crosses near the calcaneal compartment.

TREATMENT

The goal of surgical treatment of an ischemic contracture of the leg or foot is to establish a pain-free, plantigrade foot with as high a functional level as possible. Little has been written regarding correction of this debilitating problem. However, the principals of correction of the cavovarus foot have been reported and may be applied in certain cases.[14–17] The degree of deformity depends on the compartments involved. Subtle deformities can alter the weight-bearing stresses applied to the foot causing pain and effecting function. The severely malpositioned, contracted limb can result in complete loss of function, pain, and compromise of the skin and soft tissues; the latter possibly leading to chronic infection. Bracing, orthotics, and shoe modification may be a benefit in a subtle flexible deformity. However, surgical management is indicated in the more severe deformity where there is functional loss and compromise of soft tissues.

Surgical management requires a meticulous physical examination and a thorough understanding of the deforming forces and the effects these forces have had on the static and dynamic supports of the foot. The flexor hallucis longus is most commonly involved, followed by the tibialis posterior and flexor digitorum longus muscles.[18] The gastrocnemius-soleus complex is less commonly affected. Injury and subsequent contracture of these muscles can be isolated or more commonly occur in combinations involving multiple muscles or compartments.

As in the evaluation of an individual with a cavovarus alignment, determination of the driving forces must be established. The Coleman-block test may aid in differentiating the rigid varus hindfoot from one that is supple and driven by changes in forefoot position. Evaluation of foot or shank motion as well as subtalar, midfoot, and forefoot mobility will aid further in the precise determination in the structures involved.

POSTERIOR COMPARTMENT

The involvement of the superficial posterior compartment results in equinovarus deformity. Depending on the degree of deformity, this may be addressed by a simple gastrocnemius recession or Achilles tendon lengthening. Release of the deforming force can resolve both the varus and equinus deformity. In cases of severe equinus deformity with a viable deep compartment, a transfer of the flexor hallucis longus to the calcaneus or distal Achilles may be indicated to maintain plantar flexion power.

DEEP POSTERIOR COMPARTMENT

One of the authors (MDC) has had experience with two individuals demonstrating ischemic contracture involving the flexor hallucis (FHL) and flexor digitorum longus (FDL) tendons. Both patients' chief complaint was painful calluses on the pads of the great and lesser toes. Both demonstrated a tenodesis effect of the involved muscles: the digits were supple with the foot in a plantarflexed position. Passive dorsiflexion of the ankle resulted in clawing of the hallux and lesser toes. One individual was a high school student wanting to participate in sports during the current year and the other an elderly woman in poor health. Surgery consisted of exposing the flexor tendons through a posteromedial approach. The FHL and FDL tendons were divided while passively plantarflexing the foot and digits. While protecting the neurovascular bundle, a tendon stripper was used to remove the proximal portions of the tendons. The synovial lining was debrided and the sheaths sutured, collapsing the hiatus. At one year, neither patient had demonstrated recurrence. However, in cases of severe contraction and deformity, excision of the scarred muscle and descending tendon should be routine in an effort to avoid recurrence.[19]

In cases of deep posterior compartment sparing and anterior and lateral compartment weakness, the gastrocsoleus complex can be lengthened to resolve the equinus deformity. The posterior tibialis can be transferred through the interosseous membrane to the dorsum of the foot either laterally, or split medially and laterally. Whereas loss of longitudinal arch in the face of posterior tibialis transfer for Charcot-Marie-Tooth has not been observed, a viable flexor digitorum longus can be transferred to the cuneiform and function as an inverter. It has been pointed out that the spring ligament should be left intact unless the talonavicular joint is to be fused.[20]

In addition to addressing the dynamic stabilizers of the foot, structural realignment may be necessary, the concept being the creation a valgus moment about the ankle and a balanced "tripod" at the foot. In subtle deformities, dorsiflexion of the first ray may suffice to balance the foot and ankle. More severe deformities may require a biplanar, closing-wedge osteotomy that both dorsiflexes and abducts the forefoot. The hindfoot may be corrected by lateralizing the calcaneal tuberosity or by performing a closing-wedge (Dwyer) osteotomy.

RIGID DEFORMITY

Rigid plantar medial subluxation of the foot and talus in association with a fixed equinus deformity generally occurs with multicompartment involvement. This may also include flexion deformity of the digits. Surgical management in these cases would consist of excision of the scarred muscle and affected tendon. Bony realignment may be accomplished by a combination of osteotomies and arthrodeses.[16,17] Intraoperatively, the degree of correction should be assessed after sequential release of soft tissues. These include tendons, ligaments, and joint capsules; typically in that order. Depending on the degree of deformity and length of time it has existed, it may be necessary to shorten the bony elements in an effort to achieve a desired alignment. In severe long-standing contractures, it may be necessary to shorten the bony elements to restore alignment. In particular, the body or head of the talus may be contoured to reduce the tibiotalar and talonavicular joints respectively. This technique will avoid excessive tension on neurovascular structures and skin.

The lateral static constraints of the ankle must be assessed after realignment of the ankle and hindfoot. Prolonged plantar medial subluxation of the foot may cause attenuation of the lateral ankle joint capsule, necessitating repair to avoid laxity.[20]

Another concern with regard to restoration of alignment is the skin. Correction of a severely equinus or equinovarus deformity may need to be done slowly with a dynamic external fixator. In less severe cases a dynamic splint may be used or pie crusting of the skin performed. These techniques allow the skin to accommodate to the tensile forces associated with the correction.

FOOT INTRINSIC CONTRACTURE

For isolated claw toe deformities that are passively reducible, percutaneous tenotomies of both long and intrinsic flexors may be performed. The interphalangeal joint capsules may necessitate release as well. These patients should be informed of the risk of recurrence and observed. In fixed deformities of the lesser toes, a more traditional Girdlestone-Taylor procedure may be indicated. In these circumstances, one must be careful that the long flexor demonstrates a supple excursion avoiding the tenodesis effect described earlier.

POSTOPERATIVE CARE

Postoperatively, the patient should be maintained in some form of rigid support or brace for a period of 8 to 12 weeks. Supervised joint and soft tissue immobilization may be started immediately after soft tissue release, and 6 to 8 weeks after soft tissue procedures involving tendon transfers. Functional rehabilitation including range of motion, proprioception, and gait training should be initiated after radiographic evidence of bony healing when osteotomies or arthrodesis are performed.

SUMMARY

Early diagnosis and treatment of compartment syndrome of the leg or foot is invaluable in avoiding a chronic and often debilitating course. In cases where an ischemic contracture results in pain, disability, soft tissue compromise, or, as is often the case, all three of these issues, surgical intervention is indicated. Thorough physical examination of patients and their needs, and a thorough understanding of the pathomechanics as they relate to the bony structure and dynamic and static supports of the foot and ankle are paramount. These combined with a comprehensive preoperative plan and meticulous execution can often provide improved function and decrease pain in patients affected by this debilitating problem.

REFERENCES

1. Bhattacharyya T, Vrahas MS. The medical–legal aspects of compartment syndrome. J Bone Joint Surg Am 2004;86-A(4):864–8.
2. Bourne RB, Rorabeck CH. Compartment syndromes of the lower leg. Clin Orthop Relat Res 1989;240:97–104.
3. Santi MD, Botte MJ. Volkmann's ischemic contracture of the foot and ankle: evaluation and treatment of established deformity. Foot Ankle Int 1995;16(6): 368–77.
4. Mubarak SJ, Owen CA. Double-incision fasciotomy of the leg for decompression in compartment syndromes. J Bone Joint Surg Am 1977;59(2):184–7.
5. Cohen MS, Garfin SR, Hargens AR, et al. Acute compartment syndrome. Effect of dermotomy on fascial decompression in the leg. J Bone Joint Surg Br 1991;73(2): 287–90.
6. Gulli B, Templeman D. Compartment syndrome of the lower extremity. Orthop Clin North Am 1994;25(4):677–84.
7. Manoli A II. Compartment syndromes of the foot: current concepts. Foot Ankle 1990;10(6):340–4 [Review].
8. Bayer JH, Davies AP, Darrah C, et al. Calcaneal compartment syndrome after tibial fractures. Foot Ankle Int 2001;22(2):120–2.
9. Manoli A II, Weber TG. Fasciotomy of the foot: an anatomical study with special reference to release of the calcaneal compartment. Foot Ankle 1990;10(5): 267–75.
10. Myerson M, Manoli A. Compartment syndromes of the foot after calcaneal fractures. Clin Orthop Relat Res 1993;290:142–50.
11. Perry MD, Manoli A II. Foot compartment syndrome. Orthop Clin North Am 2001; 32(1):103–11.
12. Andermahr J, Helling HJ, Tsironis K, et al. Compartment syndrome of the foot. Clin Anat 2001;14(3):184–9.
13. Karlström G, Lönnerholm T, Olerud S. Cavus deformity of the foot after fracture of the tibial shaft. J Bone Joint Surg Am 1975;57(7):893–900.
14. Klaue K. Hindfoot issues in the treatment of the cavovarus foot. Foot Ankle Clin 2008;13(2):221–7.
15. Younger ASE, Hansen ST Jr. Adult cavovarus foot. J Am Acad Orthop Surg 2005; 13(5):302–15.
16. Mosier-LaClair S. Reconstruction of the varus ankle from soft-tissue procedures with osteotomy through arthrodesis. Foot Ankle Clin 2007;12(1):153–76.
17. Sullivan RJ, Aronow MS. Different faces of the triple arthrodesis. Foot Ankle Clin 2002;7(1):95–106.
18. Seddon HJ. Volkmann's ischaemia in the lower limb. J Bone Joint Surg Br 1966; 48(4):627–36.
19. Manoli A, Smith DG, Hansen ST Jr. Scarred muscle excision for the treatment of established ischemic contracture of the lower extremity. Clinical Orthopaedics and Related Research 1993;292:309–14.
20. Chilvers M, Manoli A. The subtle cavus foot and association with ankle instability and lateral foot overload. Foot Ankle Clin 2008;13(2):315–24.

Index

Note: Page numbers of article titles are in **boldface** type.

A

Achilles tendon, in tibial plafond fracture repair, 584–585
  lengthening of, for compartment syndrome, 770
Adjunctive tests, for high-energy foot and ankle trauma repair, 708–709
Allograft reconstruction, for posttraumatic talar avascular necrosis, 685–686
Amputation, for high-energy foot and ankle trauma, in limb-shortening procedures, 718–719
    limb preservation vs., 715, 718
  for posttraumatic talar avascular necrosis, 689
  for tibial plafond fractures, 588
Angle of Gissane, in intra-articular calcaneus fracture repair, 666
Ankle joint, arthrodesis of, for distal tibiofibular syndesmosis injuries, 615–616
    for posttraumatic avascular necrosis of talus, 683
  biomechanics of, in distal tibiofibular syndesmosis injuries, 614–616
  fractures of, **593–610**
    biomechanical considerations of, 593, 602
    classification of, 594
    decision-making in, 596, 598, 602–603
    in distal tibiofibular syndesmosis injuries, 616–617, 623–625
    injury patterns of, 594–597
      posteromedial variants of, 605–608
      pronation-adduction, 595, 597
        operative treatment of, 600–602
      pronation-external rotation, 595, 597
        operative treatment of, 602–603
      supination-adduction, 595–596
        operative treatment of, 600–601
      supination-external rotation, 594–595
        operative treatment of, 599–600
    malunited, reconstruction of, **737–751**
      clear space widening and, 738–739
      complexity of, 749–750
      diagnosis in, 737–738
      extra-articular deformity in, 747–749
      fibula lengthening and internal rotation in, 738–742
      management principles for, 737–738
      medial malleolus in, 744–746
      posterior malleolus in, 746–747
      radiographs of, 738, 740–741, 750
      summary overview of, 737, 750
      syndesmosis in, 741–743
      tibial plafond deformity in, 742–746
      timing of, 737–739

Foot Ankle Clin N Am 13 (2008) 773–800
doi:10.1016/S1083-7515(08)00084-3
1083-7515/08/$ – see front matter © 2008 Elsevier Inc. All rights reserved.

foot.theclinics.com

Ankle joint (*continued*)
    medial malleolus fracture with, 594–596
    operative treatment of, 598–599
        fibular length and rotation in, 596, 598–599, 602, 607
        general considerations of, 598
        internal fixation principles for, 598–599
        specific injury patterns and, 599–605
        syndesmotic fixation in, 604–605
        with posterior malleolus, 602–603
        with syndesmotic instability, 602–604
    postoperative protocols for, 607–608
    radiographic considerations of, 596, 598, 605, 607–608
    summary overview of, 593, 608
  high-energy trauma to, **705–723**. See also *High-energy trauma.*
Anterior inferior tibiofibular ligament (AITFL), in ankle biomechanics, 614
  in ankle fractures, 594–595
  in distal tibiofibular syndesmosis anatomy, 612–613
    instability related to, 614–615
  in distal tibiofibular syndesmosis injuries, 616–617, 620
    treatment of, 622–623, 625, 628
Anterior main fragment, in intra-articular calcaneus fractures, 660–661, 665–666
Anterior process calcaneus fractures, of Chopart joint, 691–692
Anterolateral approach, to tibial plafond fracture repair, 579, 581, 584–585
Anteromedial approach, modified, to tibial plafond fracture repair, 577, 579, 583
Arthritis, posttraumatic, with ankle fractures, 593
    with distal tibiofibular syndesmosis injuries, 615–616
      treatment of, 627–628
    with intra-articular calcaneus fractures, 675–676
    with Lisfranc dislocations, 699
    with talus fractures, 640, 645
Arthrodeses, ankle, for distal tibiofibular syndesmosis injuries, 615–616
    for posttraumatic avascular necrosis of talus, 683
  Blair tibiotalar, for posttraumatic avascular necrosis of talus, 684
  for Lisfranc injuries, complete vs. partial, 703
    primary, 698, 701–702
  for navicular injuries, 682, 684–685
  for posttraumatic avascular necrosis of talus, principles of, 683
    specific techniques for, 683–685
  pantalar, for posttraumatic avascular necrosis of talus, 685
  partial, for Lisfranc injuries, 703
  primary, for intra-articular calcaneus fracture repair, 673–674
    for Lisfranc injuries, 698, 701–702
  selected, for definitive reconstruction, of high-energy foot and ankle trauma, 715
  subtalar, for posttraumatic avascular necrosis of talus, 683–684
  syndesmosis, in malunited ankle fracture reconstruction, 741–743
  talonavicular, for posttraumatic avascular necrosis of talus, 684
  tibiocalcaneal, for posttraumatic avascular necrosis of talus, 684–685
  tibiofibular, for distal tibiofibular syndesmosis injuries, 627–628
  tibiotalocalcaneal, for posttraumatic avascular necrosis of talus, 684–685
  triple, for posttraumatic avascular necrosis of talus, 685
Arthroscopic debridement, of distal tibiofibular syndesmosis injuries, 623, 625, 627

Arthroscopic resection, of distal tibiofibular syndesmosis injuries, 625–627

Autograft reconstruction, vascularized, for posttraumatic talar avascular necrosis, 686

Avascular necrosis (AVN), posttraumatic, of Chopart joint, with navicular injuries, 684

        with talar head injuries, 680–681

    of talus, **753–765**

        amputation for, 689

        anatomy review of, 753–754

        arthrodesis for, 683–685

            ankle, 683

            Blair tibiotalar, 684

            pantalar, 685

            principles of, 683

            subtalar, 683–684

            talonavicular, 684

            tibiocalcaneal, 684–685

            tibiotalocalcaneal, 684–685

            triple, 685

        clinical investigations for, 680–681

        conservative treatment of, 682

        core decompression for, 682

        injury overview of, 754

        joint-sacrificing procedures for, arthrodesis as, 683–685

            total talectomy as, 682

        joint-sparing procedures for, allograft reconstruction as, 685–686

            joint replacement as, 686–687

            vascularized autograft reconstruction as, 686

        radiologic assessment of, 681–682

            nuclear imaging in, 682

            plain radiographs in, 681

        summary overview, 753, 763

        surgical reconstruction of infected, 687–688

        surgical reconstruction of noninfected with collapse, 682–687

            joint-sacrificing procedures, 682–685

            joint-sparing procedures, 685–687

        with head injuries, 680–681

Axial load, in ankle biomechanics, 614

  in Chopart injuries, 679–681, 685

  in Lisfranc injuries, 696

  in talus fractures, 643, 648

  in tibial plafond fractures, 571–572

B

Below-the-knee amputation, for high-energy foot and ankle trauma, 718–719

  for tibial plafond fractures, 588

Bimalleolar reduction clamp, for acute distal tibiofibular syndesmosis injuries, 623

Biomechanics, of ankle joint, 593, 602

    in distal tibiofibular syndesmosis injuries, 614–616

Blade plate fixation/reconstruction, of distal tibia nonunions, 730–733

Blair tibiotalar arthrodesis, for posttraumatic talar avascular necrosis, 684

Bohler approach, to tibial plafond fracture repair, 579

Bone foam, for definitive reconstruction, of high-energy foot and ankle trauma, 714
Bone grafts/grafting, for anterior process calcaneus fracture repair, 691
    for blade plate reconstruction, of distal tibia nonunions, 733
    for cuboid fracture repair, 689–690
    for distal tibiofibular syndesmosis injuries, 627–628
    for talar body fractures, 647
    for talar head fractures, 638, 640
    for talar neck fractures, 642
    for talus crush fractures, 655
    vascularized, for posttraumatic talar avascular necrosis, 686
Braces/bracing, for acute distal tibiofibular syndesmosis injuries, 621
    for compartment syndrome, 769, 771
Bridge plating, for ankle fracture repair, 600–602
    for high-energy foot and ankle trauma, 715
Brodén's view, of intra-articular calcaneus fractures, 663, 666, 668
B-type tibial pilon fracture, 583, 586–587

C

Calcaneal fractures, anterior process, 691–692
    compartment syndrome following, 768
    intra-articular, **659–678**
        CT scanning of, 661–662
        diagnostic evaluation of, 660
        fracture/dislocation patterns with, 670–673
        joint depression type, 664–671
        mechanisms of, 659–660
        nonoperative treatment of, 662
        open type, 673–674
        operative treatment of, 662–670
            3-D fluoroscopy for, 674
            combined (open/closed) technique for, 668, 671
            complications with, 674–676
            Essex-Lopresti technique for, 663–664, 668, 671
            extensile lateral approach to, 664–671
            locking plates for, 674–675
            minimally invasive technique for, 669–670, 672
            ORIF for, 673–674
            primary arthrodesis for, 673–674
        pathologic anatomy of, 659–660
        plain radiography of, 660–661
            posttraumatic arthritis of, 675–676
            Sanders type I, 663
            Sanders type IIA, 668
            Sanders type IIB, 668, 672
            Sanders type IIC, 663–664
            Sanders type III, 666, 668, 673
            Sanders type IV, 673–674
            split tongue type, 668, 671
            summary overview of, 659, 676
            tongue-type, 663–664, 669, 672

wound management for, 669, 673–674
   with high-energy foot and ankle trauma, 719
Casts/casting, of intra-articular calcaneus fractures, 674
  of tibial plafond fractures, 573
Cavus deformity, following compartment syndrome, 769–770
Center of rotation and angulation (CORA), for malunited fracture reconstruction, in extra-
  articular ankle deformity, 747–749
Chaput fragment, in tibial plafond fractures, 577, 579–581, 586
Chopart joint, amputation of, for high-energy foot and ankle trauma, 718
  fractures and dislocations of, **679–693**
    lateral column injuries with, 687–691
      anterior process calcaneus, 691–692
      cuboid, 687–691
    mechanisms of, 679
    medial column injuries with, 680–685
      cuneiform, 685–686, 688
      navicular, 681–686
      talar head, 680–681
    midfoot functional anatomy in, 680
    outcomes of, 691–692
    summary overview of, 679
    with high-energy foot and ankle trauma, 707, 711
Circulatory compromise. See *Vascular compromise.*
Claw toe deformity, following compartment syndrome, 769, 771
Clear space widening, in malunited ankle fractures, 738–739
Closed manipulation/treatment, of high-energy foot and ankle trauma, 708
  of intra-articular calcaneus fractures, 668, 671
  of talus fractures, 640–641, 649
  of tibial plafond fractures, 573, 575, 578
Closing wedge osteotomy, for malunited ankle fractures, 748–749
Coleman-block test, for compartment syndrome treatment, 770
Collision sports, distal tibiofibular syndesmosis injuries with, 616–617, 621
Combined (open/closed) technique, for intra-articular calcaneus fractures, 668, 671
Comminuted fractures, of talar body, 643–646
  of talar neck, 642
  of tibial plafond, 577, 582, 586
  with talus crush injuries, 654–655
Compartment pressures, in compartment syndrome, 767–768
Compartment syndrome, **767–772**
  causes of, 705, 767–768
  diagnosis of, 767–768
  late effects of, 767, 769
  Manoli description of, 768
  postoperative care for, 771
  sequelae of, 768
  summary overview of, 771–772
  treatment of, decompressive techniques for, 768
    deep posterior compartment in, 768, 770
    foot intrinsic contracture in, 771
    goal of, 769
    posterior compartment in, 770

Compartment (*continued*)

  rigid deformity in, 771

  salvage of ischemic, 769–771

 with high-energy foot and ankle trauma, 705, 709–710

  treatment of, 712–713

Complete arthrodesis, for Lisfranc injuries, 703

Compression fractures, of talus lateral process, 648–650

Compression plate fixation/reconstruction, for fibula lengthening, with malunited ankle fractures, 741–742

 of distal tibia nonunions, 730–733

Compression stocking, elastic, for intra-articular calcaneus fractures, 663

Conservative treatment, of posttraumatic talar avascular necrosis, 682

Constant fragment, in intra-articular calcaneus fractures, 660–661

Contracture(s), foot intrinsic, in compartment syndrome treatment, 771

 ischemic, in compartment syndrome, 767–769

  salvage treatment of, 769–771

Core decompression, for posttraumatic talar avascular necrosis, 682

Coronal deformity, with distal tibia nonunions, 726–727

Coronal plane, in ankle fractures, 596, 598

 in intra-articular calcaneus fracture repair, 666, 673

 in tibial plafond fractures, 577, 580, 588

Cotton test, for distal tibiofibular syndesmosis injuries, 623

Creeping substitution, in fracture nonunions, 725

Crush injuries, to Chopart joint, 679, 681, 685, 688

 to talus, 636–637, 697–699

CT scanning, of ankle fractures, 598, 605–606

  malunited, 740, 750

 of Chopart joint injuries, 679, 681, 683, 686, 689

 of distal tibiofibular syndesmosis injuries, 618–619, 624–625, 627

 of intra-articular calcaneus fractures, 661–663, 669, 671, 673–674

 of Lisfranc injuries, 697

 of posttraumatic talar avascular necrosis, 756, 759

 of talus fractures, 635–636, 640–641, 646–649, 651–652

 of tibial plafond fractures, 572–573, 576, 580, 584, 586

C-type tibial pilon fracture, 576–578, 583, 586–587

Cuboid joint, fractures of, 687–691

 in midfoot function, 680

Cuboid-metatarsal articulation injuries, salvage techniques for, 680, 690–691

Cultures, of distal tibia nonunions, with intramedullary nailing, 726

Cuneiform joint, fractures of, 685–686, 688

 in midfoot function, 680

"Cycle of injury," in high-energy foot and ankle trauma, 706

D

Debridement, arthroscopic, of distal tibiofibular syndesmosis injuries, 623, 625, 627

 in blade plate reconstruction, of distal tibia nonunions, 732–733

 irrigation and, of high-energy foot and ankle trauma, 707, 710, 718–719

 of talar body osteochondral fracture, 643–644

Decision making factors, for ankle fracture repair, 596, 598

  with posterior malleolus, 602–603

 for definitive reconstruction, of high-energy foot and ankle trauma, 713

for limb preservation vs. amputation, in high-energy foot and ankle trauma, 715–717
Decompression, core, for posttraumatic talar avascular necrosis, 682
  surgical, for compartment syndrome, 768
Decompressive fasciotomy, for foot compartment syndrome, 768
Deep posterior compartment, in compartment syndrome treatment, 768, 770
Definitive reconstruction/treatment, fixation techniques, internal definitive, for ankle
    fractures, 598–599
      for severe talus fractures, 652–654
        of tibial plafond fractures, 586–587
        of high-energy foot and ankle trauma, 713–716
      decision making factors for, 713
      implant selections for, 715–716
      principles for, 714
      selected fusions for, 715
      technical considerations for, 713–714
    of severe talus fractures, 652–654
    of tibial plafond fractures, 576–587
      anatomy for, 576–577, 582
      anterolateral approach to, 579, 581, 584–585
      internal fixation for, 586–587
      modified anteromedial approach to, 577, 579, 583
      posterolateral approach to, 583–585
      posteromedial approach to, 585
      reduction and fixation sequence for, 585–586
Degenerative joint disease (DJD), following Lisfranc dislocations, 699–700
  with malunited ankle fractures, 738, 743–744
Deltoid ligament, ankle stability role of, 593
  in ankle fractures, 594–595
    operative decisions based on, 596–597
    syndesmotic instability and, 603
  in distal tibiofibular syndesmosis injuries, 617, 619
    treatment of, 624–625
Diaphyseal tibia fractures, nonunions of, intramedullary nailing for, 725–730
Diastasis, with distal tibiofibular syndesmosis injuries, imaging studies of, 618–623
    treatment of, 621–628
      acute, 621–627
      chronic, 627–628
Dislocation(s), Lisfranc. See *Lisfranc injuries.*
  of Chopart joint, **679–693**
    lateral column injuries with, 687–691
      anterior process calcaneus, 691–692
      cuboid, 687–691
    mechanisms of, 679
    medial column injuries with, 680–685
      cuneiform, 685–686, 688
      navicular, 681–686
      talar head, 680–681
    midfoot functional anatomy in, 680
    outcomes of, 691–692
    summary overview of, 679
    with high-energy foot and ankle trauma, 707, 711

Dislocation (*continued*)
    of hindfoot, with high-energy foot and ankle trauma, 715
    of intra-articular calcaneus fractures, patterns of, 670–673
    of midfoot, with high-energy foot and ankle trauma, 714–716, 720
    of talus, with fractures. See *Talus, fracture management of.*
        with high-energy foot and ankle trauma, 707, 710–711
            outcomes of, 719–720
Displacement, of ankle fractures, 600
        fibula malunion and, 738, 740
    of intra-articular calcaneus fractures, 659–660, 669–670
        patterns of, 670–673
    of posterior medial talus fractures, 651
    of talus injuries, 754
    of talus lateral process fractures, 648–649
    of tibial plafond fractures, 572–573
        operative technique based on, 573–575, 583–584
Distal tibia nonunions, **725–735**
    blade plate reconstruction for, 730–733
    fine wire/ring external fixation for, 730
    intramedullary nailing for, 725–730
    summary overview of, 725, 733
Distal tibiofibular syndesmosis, injuries to, **611–633**
        anatomy of, 612–614
        functional, 611–612
    ankle biomechanics in, 614
    classification of, 619–621
    diagnosis of, 611, 617–619
    historical descriptions of, 611–612
    mechanism of, 616–617
    prevalence of, 611
    sectioning studies of instability causes, 614–616
    treatment of, 621–628
        acute injury techniques, 621–627
        chronic instability techniques, 627–628
Distal tibiofibular syndesmosis complex, anatomy of, 611–612
Distraction, for anterior process calcaneus fractures, 691–692
    for navicular injuries, 684
    for talar head injuries, 680, 683
    for talar neck fractures, 642
    simple, for high-energy foot and ankle trauma, 709
Dorsal anti-glide fixation, of ankle fractures, 599–600
Double contour sign, of posteromedial injury pattern, in ankle fractures, 605–606
Dynamic stabilizers, in compartment syndrome treatment, 770

E

Edwards and DeLee classification, of distal tibiofibular syndesmosis injuries, 619–620
    treatment studies on, 625
Equinus deformity, following compartment syndrome, 769–770
    rigid plantar medial subluxation with, 771
Espace clair (TCS), in distal tibiofibular syndesmosis injuries, 618

Essex-Lopresti technique, for intra-articular calcaneus fracture repair, 663–664, 668, 671
Examination under anesthesia, of Lisfranc injuries, 697
Extensile lateral approach, to intra-articular calcaneus fracture repair, 664–671
External fixation, in compartment syndrome treatment, 771
   in splinting, of high-energy foot and ankle trauma, 707, 709–711, 716
   of distal tibia nonunions, 727–730
   of intra-articular calcaneus fractures, 669
   of navicular injuries, 684
   of talar head injuries, 680–681, 683
   of tibial plafond fractures, 574–576, 578, 580–581
External rotation, in distal tibiofibular syndesmosis injuries, 616–617
      diagnostic applications of, 617–618
External rotation test, for distal tibiofibular syndesmosis injuries, 617–618
Extra-articular deformity, in malunited ankle fractures, reconstruction techniques for, 747–749
Extrinsic deformities, following compartment syndrome, 769

F

Fasciotomy, decompressive, for foot compartment syndrome, 768
Femoral distractor, for intramedullary nailing, of distal tibia nonunions, 726–727
Fibula, distal, in distal tibiofibular syndesmosis, 611–614
   fracture of, in distal tibiofibular syndesmosis injuries, 617, 622–623
      treatment of acute, 623–624, 627
      treatment of chronic, 625–628
    with tibial plafond fractures, 572
      ORIF of, 574–576, 578, 580–581
   in ankle biomechanics, 593, 614
   in ankle fracture repair, length and rotation of, 596, 598–599, 602, 607
      in malunited fractures, 738–742
    techniques for specific injuries, 599–603
   osteotomy of, in blade plate reconstruction, of distal tibia nonunions, 733
Fine wire/ring external fixation, of distal tibia nonunions, 730
Fixation techniques, combined open/closed, for intra-articular calcaneus fractures, 668, 671
   definitive reconstructive. See *Definitive reconstruction/treatment.*
   dorsal anti-glide, for ankle fracture repair, 599–600
   external. See *External fixation.*
   fine wire, for distal tibia nonunions, 730
   for anterior process calcaneus fractures, 691
   for cuboid fractures, 689–690
   for fusions. See *Arthrodeses.*
   for Lisfranc injuries, 698–703
   for talar body fractures, 643–645
   for talar head injuries, 680–681, 683–684
   internal. See *Internal fixation.*
      open reduction with. See *Open reduction and internal fixation (ORIF).*
   percutaneous reduction and, of distal tibiofibular syndesmosis injuries, 623
      of high-energy foot and ankle trauma, 711
      of intra-articular calcaneus fractures, 669, 672
   pin. See *Pin fixation.*
   plate. See *Plate fixation.*

Fixation (*continued*)
    ring, for distal tibia nonunions, 730
    screw. See *Screw fixation.*
    simple, of Lisfranc injuries, 698–699
    temporary, for high-energy foot and ankle trauma, 706–707
        external fixator for, 707, 709–711
      of Lisfranc injuries, 699
      of talar neck fractures, 642
    wire. See *Kirshner wires (K-wire) stabilization.*
Flexor digitorum longus (FDL) muscle/tendon, in compartment syndrome, 770
Flexor hallucis longus (FHL) muscle/tendon, in compartment syndrome, 770
Fluoroscopy, for ankle fracture repair, 599
      malunited, 745
    for definitive reconstruction, of high-energy foot and ankle trauma, 713–714
    for intra-articular calcaneus fracture repair, 663, 666, 668, 670
      3-D, 674
    for intramedullary nailing, of distal tibia nonunions, 726, 728
    for navicular injury repair, 684
    for talar head fracture repair, 639
Foot, compartment syndrome of, 768
      treatment of, 768–769
    compartments of, Manoli description of, 768
    high-energy trauma to, **705–723**. See also *High-energy trauma.*
Foot intrinsic contractures, in compartment syndrome treatment, 771
Force, in ankle fractures, 593, 602, 605
    in Lisfranc injuries, 696
    rotational, in distal tibiofibular syndesmosis injuries, 616–617
        diagnostic applications of, 617–618
      in distal tibiofibular syndesmosis instability, 614–615
      in tibial plafond fractures, 571
Fracture(s), compartment syndrome following, 768–769
    functional anatomy of, 593
    high-energy foot and ankle, **705–723**. See also *High-energy trauma.*
    in distal tibiofibular syndesmosis injuries, 616–617
      treatment of, 623–625
    of ankle joint, **593–610**
      biomechanical considerations of, 593, 602
      classification of, 594
      decision-making in, 596, 598, 602–603
      in distal tibiofibular syndesmosis injuries, 616–617, 623–625
      injury patterns of, 594–597
        posteromedial variants of, 605–608
        pronation-adduction, 595, 597
          operative treatment of, 600–602
        pronation-external rotation, 595, 597
          operative treatment of, 602–603
        supination-adduction, 595–596
          operative treatment of, 600–601
        supination-external rotation, 594–595
          operative treatment of, 599–600
      malunited, reconstruction of, **737–751**

clear space widening and, 738–739
complexity of, 749–750
diagnosis in, 737–738
extra-articular deformity in, 747–749
fibula lengthening and internal rotation in, 738–742
management principles for, 737–738
medial malleolus in, 744–746
posterior malleolus in, 746–747
radiographs of, 738, 740–741, 750
summary overview of, 737, 750
syndesmosis in, 741–743
tibial plafond deformity in, 742–746
timing of, 737–739
medial malleolus fracture with, 594–596
operative treatment of, 598–599
fibular length and rotation in, 596, 598–599, 602, 607
general considerations of, 598
internal fixation principles for, 598–599
specific injury patterns and, 599–605
syndesmotic fixation in, 604–605
with posterior malleolus, 602–603
with syndesmotic instability, 602–604
postoperative protocols for, 607–608
radiographic considerations of, 596, 598, 605, 607–608
summary overview of, 593, 608
of calcaneus, intra-articular, **659–678**
CT scanning of, 661–662
diagnostic evaluation of, 660
fracture/dislocation patterns with, 670–673
joint depression type, 664–671
mechanisms of, 659–660
nonoperative treatment of, 662
open type, 673–674
operative treatment of, 662–670
3-D fluoroscopy for, 674
combined (open/closed) technique for, 668, 671
complications with, 674–676
Essex-Lopresti technique for, 663–664, 668, 671
extensile lateral approach to, 664–671
locking plates for, 674–675
minimally invasive technique for, 669–670, 672
ORIF for, 673–674
primary arthrodesis for, 673–674
pathologic anatomy of, 659–660
plain radiography of, 660–661
posttraumatic arthritis of, 675–676
Sanders type I, 663
Sanders type IIA, 668
Sanders type IIB, 668, 672
Sanders type IIC, 663–664
Sanders type III, 666, 668, 673

Fracture (*continued*)

> Sanders type IV, 673–674
>
> split tongue type, 668, 671
>
> summary overview of, 659, 676
>
> tongue-type, 663–664, 669, 672
>
> wound management for, 669, 673–674

of Chopart joint, **679–693**

> lateral column injuries with, 687–691
>
>> anterior process calcaneus, 691–692
>>
>> cuboid, 687–691
>
> mechanisms of, 679
>
> medial column injuries with, 680–685
>
>> cuneiform, 685–686, 688
>>
>> navicular, 681–686
>>
>> talar head, 680–681
>
> midfoot functional anatomy in, 680
>
> outcomes of, 691–692
>
> summary overview of, 679
>
> with high-energy foot and ankle trauma, 707, 711

of pilon, B-type vs. C-type, 576–578, 583, 586–587

> with foot and ankle trauma, 708–709
>
> with tibial plafond fractures, 576–578, 583

of talus, **635–657**

> body, 687–692
>
> crush, 697–699
>
> general considerations for, 635–636
>
> head, 636–640, 680–681
>
> lateral process, 692–694
>
> neck, 684–687
>
> open, 696–697
>
> posterior medial aspect, 694–697
>
> summary overview of, 635, 655–656

of tibia, compartment syndrome following, 768–769

> distal nonunions of, **725–735**
>
>> blade plate reconstruction for, 730–733
>>
>> fine wire/ring external fixation for, 730
>>
>> intramedullary nailing for, 725–730
>>
>> summary overview of, 725, 733
>
> in distal tibiofibular syndesmosis injuries, treatment of acute, 624, 627
>
>> treatment of chronic, 625–628

of tibial plafond, **571–591**

> assessment of, 572–573
>
> mechanisms of, 571–572
>
> nonoperative treatment of, 573
>
> nonreconstructable, 587–588
>
> operative treatment of, 573–587
>
>> definitive (stage 2), 576–587
>>
>>> anatomy for, 576–577, 582
>>>
>>> anterolateral approach to, 579, 581, 584–585
>>>
>>> internal fixation for, 586–587
>>>
>>> modified anteromedial approach to, 577, 579, 583

      posterolateral approach to, 583–585

      posteromedial approach to, 585

      reduction and fixation sequence for, 585–586

    determinants of technique for, 573–574

    external fixation as, tibial, 574–576, 578, 580–581

    ORIF as, fibular, 574–576, 578, 580–581

      general approach to, 574, 587

    urgent (stage 1), 574–576, 578, 580–581

  outcomes of, 588–589

  physical examination of, 572

  radiographic examination of, 572–573

  rehabilitation for, 587

  summary overview of, 571–572, 589

Fracture blisters, re-epithelialization of, in high-energy foot and ankle trauma, 713

Fracture boot, for intra-articular calcaneus fractures, 663

Fragments, in intra-articular calcaneus fractures, 660–661, 663, 665–666, 669–670

  in tibial plafond fractures, 577, 579–581, 586

Frick's test, for distal tibiofibular syndesmosis injuries, 617

Functional anatomy, of ankle, 593

  of distal tibiofibular syndesmosis, 611–612

  of fibula, 593, 614

  of medial malleolus, 593

  of midfoot, 680

  of talus, 593, 635

Functional compromise, with chronic distal tibiofibular syndesmosis injuries, 627

  with compartment syndrome, 769, 771

Fusions. See *Arthrodeses.*

G

Gait, Chopart joint function in, 680

  talus function in, 635

Gastrocnemius recession, for compartment syndrome, 770

Gastrocsoleus complex, lengthening of, for compartment syndrome, 770

Grafts/grafting, bone. See *Bone grafts/grafting.*

  for posttraumatic talar avascular necrosis, 685–686

  skin, for amputation, with high-energy foot and ankle trauma, 718

Gravity stress test, for ankle fracture repair decisions, 598

H

Hardcastle classification, of Lisfranc injuries, 696–697

Hawkins classification, of talus injuries, 754

Hawkins sign, in posttraumatic talar avascular necrosis, 755

Heterotopic ossifications, following distal tibiofibular syndesmosis injuries, 627

High-energy trauma, to foot and ankle, **705–723**

    calcaneus fracture/dislocation patterns with, 670–673

    definitive reconstruction of, 713–716

    decision making factors for, 713

    implant selections for, 715–716

    principles for, 714

High-energy (*continued*)
  selected fusions for, 715
  technical considerations for, 713–714
 external fixator for splinting, 707, 709–711, 716
 initial care plan for, 705–707
 initial reduction of, 707–708
 limb preservation for, 716–719
  amputation vs., 715, 718
  decision making factors for, 715–717
  limb-shortening procedures for, 718–719
  multidisciplinary approach to, 708, 716
  objective studies of, 717
  planning for, 716–717
  scoring systems role in, 717
 limited open strategies for, 711
 outcomes of treatment, 719–720
 percutaneous techniques for, 711
 posteromedial variant injury patterns with, 605–607
 staged treatment of, 708–709
 summary overview of, 705, 720
 tibial plafond fractures with, 571–572. See also *Tibial plafond.*
 vacuum-assisted closure dressing for, 712–713
 wound management of, 712–713
  initial, 707
Hindfoot, dislocation of, with high-energy trauma, 715

  I

Ilizarov external fixator, for distal tibia fractures, nonunions with, 730
Immobilization, for acute distal tibiofibular syndesmosis injuries, 621, 624
 for intra-articular calcaneus fractures, 16, 663, 667, 673
 for talus fractures, 636, 641, 651–652
Impaction injuries, to anterior process calcaneus, 691–692
 to talar body, 647
 to talar head, 637–639
Implants, for definitive reconstruction, of high-energy foot and ankle trauma, 715–716
 for posttraumatic talar avascular necrosis, 688
 for talar body fracture repair, 647–648
 for talar head fracture repair, 638–640
 for talus lateral process fracture repair, 648
 for tibial plafond fracture repair, 579, 586–587
Incisura fibularis, of tibia, in distal tibiofibular syndesmosis anatomy, 613–614
  fracture treatment of, 623, 625
Indirect push-pull technique, for ankle fracture repair, 599
Individualized care plan, for high-energy foot and ankle trauma, **705–723**. See also *High-energy trauma.*
Infection, with distal tibia nonunions, 726–731
 with high-energy foot and ankle trauma, 708, 710–711, 720
 with posttraumatic talar avascular necrosis, 687–688
Initial care plan, for high-energy foot and ankle trauma, 705–707
Internal fixation, definitive, of severe talus fractures, 652–654
  of tibial plafond fractures, 586–587

for ankle fractures, 598–599
    open reduction with. See *Open reduction and internal fixation (ORIF).*
Internal rotation, fibula length and, in ankle fracture repair, 596, 598–599, 602, 607
        with malunited fractures, 738–742
Interosseous membrane (IOM), aponeurotic, in ankle biomechanics, 614
        in distal tibiofibular syndesmosis anatomy, 611–613
            instability related to, 614–615
        in distal tibiofibular syndesmosis injuries, 617
Interosseous tibiofibular ligament (IOL), in distal tibiofibular syndesmosis anatomy,
    612–613
        instability related to, 614–615
    in distal tibiofibular syndesmosis injuries, 617, 620
        treatment of, 628
Intra-articular fractures, of calcaneus, **659–678**
        CT scanning of, 661–662
        diagnostic evaluation of, 660
        fracture/dislocation patterns with, 670–673
        joint depression type, 664–671
        mechanisms of, 659–660
        nonoperative treatment of, 662
        open type, 673–674
        operative treatment of, 662–670
            3-D fluoroscopy for, 674
            combined (open/closed) technique for, 668, 671
            complications with, 674–676
            Essex-Lopresti technique for, 663–664, 668, 671
            extensile lateral approach to, 664–671
            locking plates for, 674–675
            minimally invasive technique for, 669–670, 672
            ORIF for, 673–674
            primary arthrodesis for, 673–674
        pathologic anatomy of, 659–660
        plain radiography of, 660–661
        posttraumatic arthritis of, 675–676
        Sanders type I, 663
        Sanders type IIA, 668
        Sanders type IIB, 668, 672
        Sanders type IIC, 663–664
        Sanders type III, 666, 668, 673
        Sanders type IV, 673–674
        split tongue type, 668, 671
        summary overview of, 659, 676
        tongue-type, 663–664, 669, 672
        wound management for, 669, 673–674
    of tibial plafond, 571, 582, 587. See also *Tibial plafond.*
Intramedullary (IM) nailing, for distal tibia nonunions, 725–730
Intrinsic deformities, following compartment syndrome, 769
Irrigation and debridement, of high-energy foot and ankle trauma, 707, 710, 718–719
Ischemia, in compartment syndrome, 767–768
Ischemic contractures, in compartment syndrome, 767–769
        salvage treatment of, 769–771

J

Johansen lag screw, for chronic distal tibiofibular syndesmosis injuries, 628
Joint depression type fractures, of calcaneus, 664–671
Joint replacement, for malunited ankle fractures, 737–738
    for posttraumatic talar avascular necrosis, 686–687
Joint-sacrificing procedures, for posttraumatic avascular necrosis, of talus, arthrodesis as, 683–685
        total talectomy as, 682
Joint-sparing procedures, for posttraumatic avascular necrosis, of talus, allograft reconstruction as, 685–686
joint replacement as, 686–687
        vascularized autograft reconstruction as, 686

K

Kirshner wires (K-wire) stabilization, for fibula lengthening, with malunited ankle fractures, 741
    of ankle fractures, 603–604
    of high-energy foot and ankle trauma, 707, 711, 713–714, 716
    of intra-articular calcaneus fractures, 665–666, 669
    of navicular injuries, 684
    of talar head fractures, 640
    of tibial plafond fractures, 580, 585–586

L

Lacerations, with high-energy foot and ankle trauma, 707, 712
Lag screw fixation, for ankle fracture repair, 600–601, 603
    for high-energy foot and ankle trauma fusion, 715
    Johansen, of chronic distal tibiofibular syndesmosis injuries, 628
    of cuneiform fractures, 686–687
    of intra-articular calcaneus fractures, 666, 673–674
Lateral column, in Chopart joint injuries, 687–691
        anterior process calcaneus fractures and, 691–692
        cuboid fractures and, 687–691
    in talar head fracture repair, 639–640
Lateral process fractures, of talus, 648–650
Lauge-Hansen classification, of ankle fractures, 594, 596, 605
    of distal tibiofibular syndesmosis injuries, 616–617
Leg, compartment syndrome of, late effects of, 769
    compartments of, Manoli description of, 768
Lengthening osteosynthesis, bifocal compression-distraction, for distal tibia nonunions, 730
Lengthening techniques, for fibula, in ankle fracture repair, 596, 598–599, 602, 607
        in malunited fractures, 738–742
        techniques for specific injuries, 599–603
Ligamentoplasty, peroneus longus, for chronic distal tibiofibular syndesmosis injuries, 626–628
Ligamentous junction, in distal tibiofibular syndesmosis, 611–614
        anatomy of, 612–614
        historical descriptions of, 611–612

Limb preservation, for high-energy foot and ankle trauma, 716–719
    amputation vs., 715, 718
    decision making factors for, 715–717
    limb-shortening procedures for, 718–719
    multidisciplinary approach to, 708, 716
    objective studies of, 717
    planning for, 716–717
    scoring systems role in, 717
Limb-shortening procedures, for high-energy foot and ankle trauma repair, 718–719
Limited open strategies, for high-energy foot and ankle trauma, 711
Lisfranc amputation, for high-energy foot and ankle trauma, 718
Lisfranc injuries, **695–704**
  anatomy of, 695–696
  classification of, 696–697
  clinical confirmation of, 697
  clinical picture of, 697
  imaging of, 697
  mechanism of, 696
  outcomes of, 718, 720
  summary overview of, 695, 703
  treatment of, 697–703
    complete ligamentous disruption, 698–703
    group descriptions in, 697
    incomplete ligamentous disruption, 698–699
Lisfranc ligament, anatomy of, 695–696
  disruption, complete vs. incomplete, 697. See also *Lisfranc injuries.*
Litigation, on compartment syndrome, 768
Load, axial. See *Axial load.*
  rotational. See *Rotational force.*
Locking plates, for fibula lengthening, with malunited ankle fractures, 741–742
  for intra-articular calcaneus fractures repair, 674–675
Low contact-dynamic compression (LC-DC)-type plate, for ankle fracture fixation, 602

M

Maisonneuve fracture, in ankle fractures, 602–603
  in distal tibiofibular syndesmosis injuries, 619, 624
Malleolus, fracture of medial, in distal tibiofibular syndesmosis injuries, 617
    treatment of, 623–625
  in ankle biomechanics, 614
  osteotomy of, in talar body fracture repair, 646
  posterior, in ankle fracture repair, 602–603
Mangled extremity severity score (MESS), of high-energy foot and ankle trauma, 717
Manoli description, of foot compartments, 768
Marti-Weber classification, of talus injuries, 754
Medial column, in Chopart joint injuries, 680–685
    cuneiform fractures and, 685–686, 688
    navicular, 681–686
    talar head, 680–681
  in talar head fracture repair, 639–640
  in talus crush fracture repair, 655

Medial malleolus, fracture of, in distal tibiofibular syndesmosis injuries, 617
        treatment of, 623–625
    functional anatomy of, 593
    in ankle fractures, 594–596
        malunited, reconstruction for, 744–746
    in talar neck fracture repair, 641–642
    in tibial plafond fracture repair, 584–586
Metadiaphyseal alignment, in tibial plafond fracture repair, 580–581, 587–588
Metaphyseal tibia fractures, nonunions of, external fixation for, 730
Metatarsals, in Lisfranc injuries, 695
    in midfoot function, 680
Midfoot, columns of, in Lisfranc injuries, 695–697
    dislocation of, with high-energy trauma, 714–716, 720
    functional anatomy of, 680
Minimally invasive technique, for intra-articular calcaneus fracture repair, 669–670, 672
Modified anteromedial approach, to tibial plafond fracture repair, 577, 579, 583
MRI scanning, of distal tibiofibular syndesmosis injuries, 619
    of Lisfranc injuries, 697
    of posttraumatic talar avascular necrosis, 756
Multidisciplinary approach, to high-energy foot and ankle trauma repair, 708, 716
Muscles, in compartment syndrome, contracture of, 769–770
        necrosis of, 767–768
        removal of scarred, 770–771
Myocutaneous flap, in limb-shortening procedures, for high-energy foot and ankle trauma,
    718

    N

Nailing, intramedullary, for distal tibia nonunions, 725–730
Navicular injuries, of Chopart joint, 681–686
Navicular motion, in midfoot function, 680
Nerves, damage to, in compartment syndrome, 767–769
        with high-energy foot and ankle trauma, 707, 717
Nonoperative treatment, of intra-articular calcaneus fractures, 662
    of tibial plafond fractures, 573
Nonreconstructable fractures, of tibial plafond, 587–588
Nonunions, of distal tibial fractures, **725–735**
        blade plate reconstruction for, 730–733
        fine wire/ring external fixation for, 730
        intramedullary nailing for, 725–730
        summary overview of, 725, 733
Nuclear imaging, of distal tibiofibular syndesmosis injuries, 618–619
    of Lisfranc injuries, 697
Nutrition, high-energy foot and ankle trauma repair and, 708, 717

    O

Objective data, for limb preservation vs. amputation decision, in high-energy foot and ankle
    trauma, 717
Open fractures, of calcaneus, intra-articular, 673–674
    of talus, 696–697

Open reduction and internal fixation (ORIF), of ankle fractures, 600
    posteromedial variant injury pattern and, 606–608
  of Chopart injuries, 691
  of cuboid fractures, 690
  of distal tibiofibular syndesmosis injuries, 623
  of intra-articular calcaneus fractures, 673–674
  of Lisfranc injuries, 698–703
  of talar body fractures, 645–648
  of talar head injuries, 680, 683
  of talus neck fractures, 640–641
  of tibial plafond fractures, fibular, 574–576, 578, 580–581
    general approach to, 574, 587
    outcomes of, 588–589
Open strategies, limited, for high-energy foot and ankle trauma, 711
Orthopaedic Trauma Association (OTA), tibial plafond fracture classification of, 576–577
Os trigonum fracture, of posterior medial talus, 694–697
Osteoarthrosis, following Lisfranc dislocations, 699, 703
  following navicular injuries, 682
Osteochondral allografts, for posttraumatic talar avascular necrosis, 685–686
Osteochondral fracture, of talus, 643–644
Osteomyelitis. See *Infection.*
Osteopenia, in malunited ankle fractures, 738, 742–743
Osteosynthesis, bifocal compression-distraction lengthening, for distal tibia nonunions, 730
Osteotomy(ies), closing wedge, for malunited ankle fractures, 748–749
  fibular, for lengthening, with malunited ankle fractures, 740–742
    in blade plate reconstruction, of distal tibia nonunions, 733
  in compartment syndrome treatment, 770
  malleolus, in talar body fracture repair, 646
  tibial, in talar body fracture repair, 646–647
    lateral, in malunited ankle fracture reconstruction, 742–746

P

Pain, in compartment syndrome diagnosis, 767–769
  with distal tibiofibular syndesmosis injuries, 617–618
Pantalar arthrodesis, for posttraumatic talar avascular necrosis, 685
Parasthesias, in compartment syndrome diagnosis, 767
Partial arthrodesis, for Lisfranc injuries, 703
Partial articular injuries, of tibial plafond, 576
Percutaneous reduction and fixation, of distal tibiofibular syndesmosis injuries, 623
  of high-energy foot and ankle trauma, 711
  of intra-articular calcaneus fractures, 669, 672
Periarticular tibia fractures, nonunions of, blade plate reconstruction for, 730–733
Peroneal nerve, in acute distal tibiofibular syndesmosis injuries, 623
  in compartment syndrome, 768
Peroneal tendons, in intra-articular calcaneus fracture repair, 667, 671
Peroneus longus ligamentoplasty, for chronic distal tibiofibular syndesmosis injuries, 626–628
Physical examination, of tibial plafond fractures, 572
Physical therapy, for acute distal tibiofibular syndesmosis injuries, 621
  for intra-articular calcaneus fractures, 663, 667, 674
  for tibial plafond fractures, 573, 587

Pilon, fractures of, B-type vs. C-type, 576–578, 583, 586–587
    nonreconstructable, 587–588
    operative outcomes of, 588–589
    with high-energy foot and ankle trauma, 708–709
    with tibial plafond fractures, 576–578, 583
Pin fixation, of intra-articular calcaneus fractures, 665–666, 668–669, 671
    of talar body fractures, 647–648
    of talar head fractures, 640
    of talar neck fractures, 642
    of tibial plafond fractures, 575–578, 581, 585
Pin tract infection, with external fixation, of distal tibia fractures, 727–730
Plafond, tibial, anatomy of, 576–577, 582
        fractures of, **571–591**. See also Tibial plafond.
Plafondplasty, in malunited ankle fracture reconstruction, 742–746
Plantar joint, in talar head fractures, 637–638
Plantar ligaments, in cuboid fractures, 687
    in Lisfranc injuries, 695–697
        complete disruption and, 698–703
        incomplete disruption and, 698–699
Plantar medial subluxation, with equinus deformity, following compartment syndrome, 771
Plate fixation, blade, of distal tibia nonunions, 730–733
    for fibula lengthening, with malunited ankle fractures, 741–742
    for high-energy foot and ankle trauma, 715–716
    of ankle fractures, 599–604
    of cuboid fractures, 689–690
    of cuneiform fractures, 686, 688–690
    of intra-articular calcaneus fractures, 666–667, 669, 674–675
    of navicular injuries, 684
    of talar head injuries, 680–681
    of tibial plafond fractures, 577, 580, 586–587
PMMA cement block, for posttraumatic talar avascular necrosis, 688
"Positive wrinkle sign," in high-energy foot and ankle trauma, 713
Posterior compartment, in compartment syndrome treatment, 770
Posterior inferior tibiofibular ligament (PITFL), in ankle biomechanics, 614
    in ankle fractures, 594–595
    in distal tibiofibular syndesmosis anatomy, 612–613
        instability related to, 614–615
    in distal tibiofibular syndesmosis injuries, 617
        treatment of, 628
Posterior main fragment, in intra-articular calcaneus fractures, 660–661
Posterior malleolus, in ankle fracture repair, 602–603
        malunited, reconstruction for, 746–747
Posterior medial talus fractures, 694–697
Posterior tibialis tendon, in compartment syndrome, 770
Posterolateral approach, to tibial plafond fracture repair, 583–585
Posteromedial approach, to distal tibia nonunions, 732–733
    to tibial plafond fracture repair, 585
Posteromedial variants, of ankle fracture injuries, 605–608
Primary arthrodesis, for intra-articular calcaneus fracture repair, 673–674
    for Lisfranc injuries, 698, 701–702
Pronation-adduction injury pattern, in ankle fractures, 595, 597

operative treatment of, 600–602
Pronation-external rotation injury pattern, in ankle fractures, 595, 597
    operative treatment of, 602–603
Prostheses, for amputation, with high-energy foot and ankle trauma, 718–719
    talar, for posttraumatic avascular necrosis, 686–687
Proximal tibiofibular syndesmosis, in distal tibiofibular syndesmosis anatomy, 611–612
Psychological aspects, of high-energy foot and ankle trauma, 708, 716–717
Push-pull technique, indirect, for ankle fracture repair, 599

R

Radiographs, of ankle fractures, 596, 598, 605, 607–608
        malunited, reconstruction and, 738, 740–741, 750
    of Chopart joint injuries, 679, 681, 685, 688–689
    of distal tibiofibular syndesmosis injuries, 618–624
    of intra-articular calcaneus fracture, 660–661
    of intramedullary nailing, for distal tibia nonunions, 726, 728–729
    of Lisfranc injuries, 696–697, 699–701
    of posttraumatic talar avascular necrosis, 681–682, 755
    of talus fractures, 635–636, 639–641, 648–649, 651
    of tibial plafond fractures, 572, 580, 582, 584
Range-of-motion exercises. See *Physical therapy.*
Realignment, structural, in compartment syndrome treatment, 770–771
Reconstruction techniques, surgical, definitive. See also *Definitive
    reconstruction/treatment.*
        for high-energy foot and ankle trauma, 691, 713–716
        for severe talus fractures, 652–654
        for tibial plafond fractures, 576–587
    for chronic distal tibiofibular syndesmosis injuries, 627–628
    for crush fractures, of talus, 654–655
    for cuboid fractures, 688
    for cuboid-metatarsal articulations, 680, 690–691
    for malunited ankle fractures, **737–751**
        clear space widening and, 738–739
        complexity of, 749–750
        diagnosis in, 737–738
        extra-articular deformity in, 747–749
        fibula lengthening and internal rotation in, 738–742
        management principles for, 737–738
        medial malleolus in, 744–746
        posterior malleolus in, 746–747
        radiographs of, 738, 740–741, 750
        summary overview of, 737, 750
        syndesmosis in, 741–743
        tibial plafond deformity in, 742–746
        timing of, 737–739
    for navicular injuries, 684
    for posttraumatic avascular necrosis of talus, infected, 687–688
        noninfected with collapse, 682–687
            joint-sacrificing procedures, 682–685
            joint-sparing procedures, 685–687
    for talar body fracture, 647–648

Reconstruction (*continued*)
  for talar head injuries, 680
  grafting for. See *specific grafts.*
  secondary, for malunited ankle fractures, 737
Reduction clamp, bimalleolar, for acute distal tibiofibular syndesmosis injuries, 623
  for navicular injury repair, 684
Reduction techniques, closed. See *Closed manipulation/treatment.*
  for high-energy foot and ankle trauma, initial, 707–708
  for navicular injuries, of Chopart joint, 681–682
  for posterior medial talus fractures, 651, 653
  for talar head fracture, 637–638
  for talar neck fractures, 642
  for tibial plafond fractures, fixation sequence with, 585–586
    force vectors in, 580
  open. See *Open reduction and internal fixation (ORIF).*
  percutaneous, and fixation, for distal tibiofibular syndesmosis injuries, 623
      for high-energy foot and ankle trauma, 711
      for intra-articular calcaneus fractures, 669, 672
Re-epithelialization, of fracture blisters, in high-energy foot and ankle trauma, 713
Rehabilitation, for acute distal tibiofibular syndesmosis injuries, 621–623
  for high-energy foot and ankle trauma, 716–717
  for intra-articular calcaneus fractures, 667, 673–674
  for talar head injuries, 681
  for talus fractures, 636
  for tibial plafond fractures, 573, 587
Resection, arthroscopic, of distal tibiofibular syndesmosis injuries, 625–627
Return to activity, following distal tibiofibular syndesmosis injuries, 621–622
  following Lisfranc injury repair, 699, 701–702
Rhabdomyolysis, in compartment syndrome, 767
RICE therapy, for acute distal tibiofibular syndesmosis injuries, 621
Rigid deformity, in compartment syndrome treatment, 771
Ring fixation, external, of distal tibia nonunions, 730
Rotational force, external, in distal tibiofibular syndesmosis injuries, 616–617
      diagnostic applications of, 617–618
  in distal tibiofibular syndesmosis instability, 614–615
  in tibial plafond fractures, 571
  internal, fibula length and, in ankle fracture repair, 596, 598–599, 602, 607
    in malunited ankle fractures, 738–742

S

Sagittal plane, in ankle fractures, 596
  in intra-articular calcaneus fracture repair, 666–668
  in tibial plafond fractures, 577, 580, 588
Salvage techniques, for chronic distal tibiofibular syndesmosis injuries, 627–628
  for crush fractures, of talus, 654–655
  for cuboid fractures, 688
  for cuboid-metatarsal articulation, 680, 690–691
  for high-energy foot and ankle trauma, 716–719
    amputation vs., 715, 718
    decision making factors for, 715–717

limb-shortening procedures for, 718–719
multidisciplinary approach to, 708, 716
objective studies of, 717
planning for, 716–717
scoring systems role in, 717
for ischemic contractures, in compartment syndrome, 769–771
for malunited ankle fractures, 737
for navicular injuries, 684
for posttraumatic avascular necrosis of talus, infected, 687–688
noninfected with collapse, 682–687
joint-sacrificing procedures, 682–685
joint-sparing procedures, 685–687
for talar body fracture, 647–648
for talar head injuries, 680
grafting for. See *specific grafts.*
Sanders type I intra-articular fractures, of calcaneus, 663
Sanders type IIA intra-articular fractures, of calcaneus, 668
Sanders type IIB intra-articular fractures, of calcaneus, 668, 672
Sanders type IIC intra-articular fractures, of calcaneus, 663–664
Sanders type III intra-articular fractures, of calcaneus, 666, 668, 673
Sanders type IV intra-articular fractures, of calcaneus, 673–674
Schanz pin, for definitive reconstruction, of high-energy foot and ankle trauma, 714
for intra-articular calcaneus fracture repair, 665–666, 668–669, 671
for tibial plafond fracture fixation, 575–577, 581, 585
Scoring systems, for high-energy foot and ankle trauma repair, 691, 717
Screw fixation, for high-energy foot and ankle trauma fusion, 715
of ankle fractures, 600–601, 603–604
of cuneiform fractures, 686–687
of distal tibiofibular syndesmosis injuries, 615–616, 619
acute, 623–625
chronic, 627–628
of intra-articular calcaneus fractures, 663–667, 669, 673–674
of Lisfranc injuries, 699–700, 702
of talar body fractures, 648
of talar head fractures, 638–641, 680
of talar neck fractures, 642–643
of tibial plafond fractures, 580, 586–588
Sepsis, with high-energy foot and ankle trauma, 708, 710–711, 720
Shear fractures, of ankle joint, 605
of talar body, 643–644
of talar neck, 636–637
treatment of, 640–641
"Shenton's line of the ankle," 596
Simple fixation, of Lisfranc injuries, 698–699
Sinus tarsi approach, to talus lateral process fracture repair, 648, 650
Skeletal stabilization, of high-energy foot and ankle trauma, external fixator for, 707,
709–711, 716
initial, 705–707
staged, 708–709
Skin grafts/grafting, for amputation, with high-energy foot and ankle trauma, 718
"Snow boarder's fracture," 648

Soft tissue trauma, compartment syndrome following, 705, 767–768
    late effects of, 769
    rigid deformity with, 771
  in high-energy foot and ankle trauma, 705–706
    definitive reconstruction and, 715
    limb preservation and, 718–719
    outcomes of, 719–720
    scoring system for, 717
    staged treatment of, 708–709, 711
    tibial plafond fractures and, 571–573, 586–587
    wound management for, 712
  to Chopart joint, 679, 692
  with talus fractures, 652–655
Splints/splinting, in tibial plafond fracture rehabilitation, 587
  of high-energy foot and ankle trauma, 707, 709–711, 716
  of intra-articular calcaneus fractures, 663, 667
  postoperative, in ankle fracture repair, 607
Split tongue intra-articular fractures, of calcaneus, 668, 671
Squeeze test, for distal tibiofibular syndesmosis injuries, 617
Stabilization test, for distal tibiofibular syndesmosis injuries, 618
Stage 1 (urgent) treatment, of tibial plafond fractures, 574–576, 578, 580–581
Stage 2 treatment. See *Definitive reconstruction/treatment.*
Staged treatment, of high-energy foot and ankle trauma, 708–709
  of malunited ankle fractures, 737–738
Subluxation, talonavicular, with talar head fractures, 636, 639
Subtalar joint, arthrodesis of, for posttraumatic talar avascular necrosis, 683–684
  in talar body fracture repair, 645
  in talus crush fracture repair, 654–655
  in talus lateral process fracture repair, 648, 650–652
Superolateral fragment, in intra-articular calcaneus fractures, 660–661, 666, 670
Superomedial fragment, in intra-articular calcaneus fractures, 660–661
Supination-adduction injury pattern, in ankle joint fractures, 595–596
    operative treatment of, 600–601
Supination-external rotation injury pattern, in ankle fractures, 594–595
    operative treatment of, 599–600
Surgical decompression, core, for posttraumatic talar avascular necrosis, 682
  for compartment syndrome, 768
Surgical reconstruction. See *Reconstruction techniques.*
Sustentacular fragment, in intra-articular calcaneus fractures, 660–661
Syme amputation, for high-energy foot and ankle trauma, 718
Syndesmosis, arthrodesis of, in malunited ankle fracture reconstruction, 741–743
  distal tibiofibular, injuries to, **611–633**
      anatomy of, 612–614
      functional, 611–612
    ankle biomechanics in, 614
    classification of, 619–621
    diagnosis of, 611, 617–619
    historical descriptions of, 611–612
    mechanism of, 616–617
    prevalence of, 611
    sectioning studies of instability causes, 614–616

treatment of, 621–628
   acute injury techniques, 621–627
   chronic instability techniques, 627–628
fixation of, in ankle fracture repair, 603–605
   controversies in, 604–605
   malunited, 741–743
fusion of, in malunited ankle fracture repair, 741–743
instability of, with ankle fractures, 602–604
Syndesmosis complex, in distal tibiofibular anatomy, 611–612

T

Talar body, fractures of, 687–692
   AVN risks with, 754
Talar dome, lateral access to, in talar body fracture repair, 646–647
Talar head, fractures of, 636–640
   in Chopart joint injuries, 680–681
Talar lateral process, fractures of, 692–694
Talar neck, fractures of, 684–687
Talectomy, total, for posttraumatic avascular necrosis, 682
Talonavicular joint, arthrodesis of, for posttraumatic talar avascular necrosis, 684
   dislocations of, trauma causing, 680–681
      with talar head fractures, 636, 639
   in talus crush fracture repair, 654–655
Talus, anatomy of, 753–754
   functional, 593, 635
   dislocation of, with high-energy foot and ankle trauma, 707, 710–711
      outcomes of, 719–720
   fracture management of, **635–657**
      crush, 697–699
      general considerations for, 635–636
      of body, 687–692, 754
      of head, 636–640, 680–681
      of lateral process, 692–694
      of neck, 684–687
      of posterior medial aspect, 694–697
      open, 696–697
      summary overview of, 635, 655–656
   in ankle biomechanics, 614
   in distal tibiofibular syndesmosis injuries, 616
   in midfoot function, 680
   injuries to, overview of, 754
   posttraumatic avascular necrosis of, **753–765**
      amputation for, 689
      anatomy review of, 753–754
      arthrodesis for, 683–685
         ankle, 683
         Blair tibiotalar, 684
         pantalar, 685
         principles of, 683
         subtalar, 683–684

Talus (*continued*)
    talonavicular, 684
    tibiocalcaneal, 684–685
    tibiotalocalcaneal, 684–685
    triple, 685
  clinical investigations for, 680–681
  conservative treatment of, 682
  core decompression for, 682
  injury overview of, 754
  joint-sacrificing procedures for, arthrodesis as, 683–685
    total talectomy as, 682
  joint-sparing procedures for, allograft reconstruction as, 685–686
    joint replacement as, 686–687
    vascularized autograft reconstruction as, 686
  radiologic assessment of, 681–682
    nuclear imaging in, 682
    plain radiographs in, 681
  summary overview, 753, 763
  surgical reconstruction of infected, 687–688
  surgical reconstruction of noninfected with collapse, 682–687
    joint-sacrificing procedures, 682–685
    joint-sparing procedures, 685–687
  with head injuries, 680–681
Tarsometatarsal (TMT) joint, in Lisfranc injuries, 695–696, 702
Temporary fixation, for high-energy foot and ankle trauma, 706–707, 716
    external fixator for, 707, 709–711
  of Lisfranc injuries, 699
  of talar neck fractures, 642
Temporization, of high-energy foot and ankle trauma, 706–707, 709–711, 716
Tenotomy(ies), in compartment syndrome treatment, 771
Tension band constructs, for ankle fracture repair, 600
Tibia, distal, fractures of, **571–591**. See also *Tibial plafond.*
    nonunions of, **725–735**. See also *Nonunions.*
    in distal tibiofibular syndesmosis, 611–614
  fractures of, compartment syndrome following, 768–769
    distal, **571–591**. See also *Tibial plafond.*
    nonunions of, **725–735**. See also *Nonunions.*
    distal nonunions of, **725–735**
      blade plate reconstruction for, 730–733
      fine wire/ring external fixation for, 730
      intramedullary nailing for, 725–730
      summary overview of, 725, 733
    in distal tibiofibular syndesmosis injuries, 611
      treatment of acute, 624, 627
      treatment of chronic, 625–628
  in ankle biomechanics, 614
  lateral osteotomy of, in malunited ankle fracture reconstruction, 742–746
  osteotomies of, in talar body fracture repair, 646–647
Tibial plafond, anatomy of, 576–577, 582
  deformity of, in malunited ankle fractures, reconstruction of, 742–746
  fractures of, **571–591**

assessment of, 572–573
mechanisms of, 571–572
nonoperative treatment of, 573
nonreconstructable, 587–588
operative treatment of, 573–587
    definitive (stage 2), 576–587
        anatomy for, 576–577, 582
        anterolateral approach to, 579, 581, 584–585
        internal fixation for, 586–587
        modified anteromedial approach to, 577, 579, 583
        posterolateral approach to, 583–585
        posteromedial approach to, 585
        reduction and fixation sequence for, 585–586
    determinants of technique for, 573–574
    external fixation as, tibial, 574–576, 578, 580–581
    ORIF as, fibular, 574–576, 578, 580–581
        general approach to, 574, 587
    urgent (stage 1), 574–576, 578, 580–581
outcomes of, 588–589
physical examination of, 572
radiographic examination of, 572–573
rehabilitation for, 573, 587
summary overview of, 571–572, 589
Tibiocalcaneal arthrodesis, for posttraumatic talar avascular necrosis, 684–685
Tibiofibular arthrodesis, for distal tibiofibular syndesmosis injuries, 627–628
Tibiofibular overlap (TFO), in distal tibiofibular syndesmosis injuries, 618
Tibiofibular syndesmosis, distal injuries to, **611–633**. See also Distal
    tibiofibular syndesmosis.
Tibiofibular synostosis, in distal tibiofibular syndesmosis injuries, 627
Tibiotalar joint, Blair arthrodesis of, for posttraumatic talar avascular necrosis, 684
    in posterior medial talus fractures, 695–696
    in talar body fracture repair, 645
    in talus crush fracture repair, 655
    in tibial plafond fractures, 573–574
Tibiotalocalcaneal (TTC) arthrodesis, for posttraumatic talar avascular necrosis,
    684–685
Tongue fragment, in intra-articular calcaneus fractures, 660–661, 663–664
Tongue-type intra-articular fractures, of calcaneus, 663–664, 669, 672
Translation, as ankle fracture mechanism, 593
Transmetatarsal amputation, for high-energy foot and ankle trauma, 718
Transtibial amputation, for high-energy foot and ankle trauma, 718–719
Transverse tibiofibular ligament (TTFL), in distal tibiofibular syndesmosis anatomy,
    612–613
        instability related to, 614–615
Trauma, ankle joint fracture injury patterns from, 594–597
        posteromedial variants of, 605–608
    high-energy, Chopart fractures and dislocations with, **679–693**. See also Chopart joint.
        to foot and ankle, **705–723**. See also High-energy trauma.
    soft tissue, compartment syndrome following, 767–768
Triple arthrodesis, for posttraumatic talar avascular necrosis, 685

U

Urgent (stage 1) treatment, of tibial plafond fractures, 574–576, 578, 580–581

V

Vacuum-assisted closure (VAC) dressing, for high-energy foot and ankle trauma, 712–713
    for intra-articular calcaneus fractures, 674
Valgus deformity, in malunited ankle fractures, 742–746
Varus deformity, following compartment syndrome, 769–770
      rigid plantar deformity with, 771
    in malunited ankle fractures, 742–746, 748
Vascular compromise, in compartment syndrome, 767–768
    with high-energy foot and ankle trauma, 707, 710, 718
      measurement of, 717
      tibial plafond fractures and, 572
    with navicular injuries, of Chopart joint, 682, 684
Vascularized autograft reconstruction, for posttraumatic talar avascular necrosis, 686
Volkmann fragment, in tibial plafond fractures, 577, 580

W

"Waiting period," for high-energy foot and ankle trauma repair, 708–709
Weight bearing, with ankle fractures, 598, 607–608
    with cuboid fractures, 688
    with distal tibia nonunions, and intramedullary nailing, 726–727
    with distal tibiofibular syndesmosis injuries, 624, 627
    with intra-articular calcaneus fractures, 663, 667, 673
    with Lisfranc injuries, 696–697, 700–701
    with navicular injuries, 684
    with posttraumatic talar avascular necrosis, 682
    with talus fractures, 636, 641, 643, 648–649, 652
    with tibial plafond fractures, 571, 573, 587
West Point Ankle Grading System, for distal tibiofibular syndesmosis injuries, 620
Wire fixation. See *Kirshner wires (K-wire) stabilization.*
Wire/ring external fixation, fine, of distal tibia nonunions, 730
Wound closure, delay of, in high-energy foot and ankle trauma, 707, 711–712
    for open talus fractures, 652–653
    for tibial plafond fractures, 579
Wound dehiscence, in intra-articular calcaneus fracture repair, 674
Wound healing, in intra-articular calcaneus fracture repair, 674
Wound management, of high-energy foot and ankle trauma, 712–713
      initial, 707
      staged, 708–709
      tibial plafond fractures and, 571–572, 587–588
      VAC dressing for, 712–713
    of intra-articular calcaneus fractures, 669, 673–674
    of severe talus fractures, 652–654

Moving?

Make sure your subscription moves with you!

To notify us of your new address, find your **Clinics Account Number** (located on your mailing label above your name), and contact customer service at:

E-mail: elspcs@elsevier.com

800-654-2452 (subscribers in the U.S. & Canada)
314-453-7041 (subscribers outside of the U.S. & Canada)

Fax number: 314-523-5170

Elsevier Periodicals Customer Service
11830 Westline Industrial Drive
St. Louis, MO 63146

*To ensure uninterrupted delivery of your subscription, please notify us at least 4 weeks in advance of move.

United States Postal Service

Statement of Ownership, Management, and Circulation
(All Periodicals Publications Except Requestor Publications)

1. Publication Title	2. Publication Number	3. Filing Date
Foot and Ankle Clinics	0 1 6 - 3 6 8	9/15/08

4. Issue Frequency	5. Number of Issues Published Annually	6. Annual Subscription Price
Mar, Jun, Sep, Dec	4	$209.00

7. Complete Mailing Address of Known Office of Publication (Not printer) (Street, city, county, state, and ZIP+4)

Elsevier Inc.
360 Park Avenue South
New York, NY 10010-1710

Contact Person
Stephen Bushing
Telephone (Include area code)
215-239-3688

8. Complete Mailing Address of Headquarters or General Business Office of Publisher (Not printer)

Elsevier Inc., 360 Park Avenue South, New York, NY 10010-1710

9. Full Names and Complete Mailing Addresses of Publisher, Editor, and Managing Editor (Do not leave blank)

Publisher (Name and complete mailing address)

John Schrefler, Elsevier, Inc., 1600 John F. Kennedy Blvd. Suite 1800, Philadelphia, PA 19103-2899

Editor (Name and complete mailing address)

Deb Dellapena, Elsevier, Inc., 1600 John F. Kennedy Blvd. Suite 1800, Philadelphia, PA 19103-2899

Managing Editor (Name and complete mailing address)

Catherine Bewick, Elsevier, Inc., 1600 John F. Kennedy Blvd. Suite 1800, Philadelphia, PA 19103-2899

10. Owner (Do not leave blank. If the publication is owned by a corporation, give the name and address of the corporation immediately followed by the names and addresses of all stockholders owning or holding 1 percent or more of the total amount of stock. If not owned by a corporation, give the names and addresses of the individual owners. If owned by a partnership or other unincorporated firm, give its name and address as well as those of each individual owner. If the publication is published by a nonprofit organization, give its name and address.)

Full Name	Complete Mailing Address
Wholly owned subsidiary of	4520 East-West Highway
Reed/Elsevier, US holdings	Bethesda, MD 20814

11. Known Bondholders, Mortgagees, and Other Security Holders Owning or Holding 1 Percent or More of Total Amount of Bonds, Mortgages, or Other Securities. If none, check box ☐ None

Full Name	Complete Mailing Address
N/A	

12. Tax Status (For completion by nonprofit organizations authorized to mail at nonprofit rates) (Check one)
The purpose, function, and nonprofit status of this organization and the exempt status for federal income tax purposes:
☐ Has Not Changed During Preceding 12 Months
☐ Has Changed During Preceding 12 Months (Publisher must submit explanation of change with this statement)

PS Form 3526, September 2006 (Page 1 of 3 (Instructions Page 3)) PSN 7530-01-000-9931 PRIVACY NOTICE: See our Privacy policy in www.usps.com

---

13. Publication Title		14. Issue Date for Circulation Data Below
Foot and Ankle Clinics		September 2008

15. Extent and Nature of Circulation			Average No. Copies Each Issue During Preceding 12 Months	No. Copies of Single Issue Published Nearest to Filing Date
a. Total Number of Copies (Net press run)			1600	1600
b. Paid Circulation (By Mail and Outside the Mail)	(1)	Mailed Outside-County Paid Subscriptions Stated on PS Form 3541. (Include paid distribution above nominal rate, advertiser's proof copies, and exchange copies)	902	893
	(2)	Mailed In-County Paid Subscriptions Stated on PS Form 3541 (Include paid distribution above nominal rate, advertiser's proof copies, and exchange copies)		
	(3)	Paid Distribution Outside the Mails Including Sales Through Dealers and Carriers, Street Vendors, Counter Sales, and Other Paid Distribution Outside USPS®	179	171
	(4)	Paid Distribution by Other Classes Mailed Through the USPS (e.g. First-Class Mail®)		
c. Total Paid Distribution (Sum of 15b (1), (2), (3), and (4))		▶	1081	1064
d. Free or Nominal Rate Distribution (By Mail and Outside the Mail)	(1)	Free or Nominal Rate Outside-County Copies Included on PS Form 3541	52	50
	(2)	Free or Nominal Rate In-County Copies Included on PS Form 3541		
	(3)	Free or Nominal Rate Copies Mailed at Other Classes Mailed Through the USPS (e.g. First-Class Mail)		
	(4)	Free or Nominal Rate Distribution Outside the Mail (Carriers or other means)		
e. Total Free or Nominal Rate Distribution (Sum of 15d (1), (2), (3) and (4))		▶	52	50
f. Total Distribution (Sum of 15c and 15e)		▶	1133	1114
g. Copies not Distributed (See instructions to publishers #4 (page #3))		▶	467	486
h. Total (Sum of 15f and g)			1600	1600
i. Percent Paid (15c divided by 15f times 100)		▶	95.41%	95.51%

16. Publication of Statement of Ownership

☐ If the publication is a general publication, publication of this statement is required. Will be printed in the **December 2008** issue of this publication. ☐ Publication not required.

17. Signature and Title of Editor, Publisher, Business Manager, or Owner

Stephen Bushing – Executive Director of Subscription Services

Date: September 15, 2008

I certify that all information furnished on this form is true and complete. I understand that anyone who furnishes false or misleading information on this form or who omits material or information requested on the form may be subject to criminal sanctions (including fines and imprisonment) and/or civil sanctions (including civil penalties).

PS Form 3526, September 2006 (Page 2 of 3)